Proceedings:

AIDS Prevention and Services Workshop

February 15–16, 1990
Washington, D.C.

Vivian E. Fransen, Editor

A Publication of The Robert Wood Johnson Foundation Communications Office
Thomas P. Gore II, Vice President for Communications
Contributing Editors: Johanna Van Wert, Victoria D. Weisfeld
Production Coordinator: Joan Hollendonner

Princeton, New Jersey
June 1990

1

This Workshop on AIDS Prevention and Services was conducted by the National Health Policy Forum through a grant from The Robert Wood Johnson Foundation. The Workshop brought together selected Foundation grantees in the areas of AIDS health services, prevention and research with federal health policymakers in an effort to provide information about what these grantees had learned through their efforts to address the epidemic.

The National Health Policy Forum is a nonpartisan education and information exchange for senior federal health policymakers, including White House and congressional staff and others in the many agencies responsible for health programs and delivery. Guided by a steering committee of key congressional and regulatory health officials, it has served for more than 18 years to provide frequent contact with leaders from the corporate, provider, and research communities. Funded primarily through foundation grants and corporate contributions, the program is widely known and highly regarded for its ability to interpret issues and provide a framework for addressing today's health policy dilemmas.

The Robert Wood Johnson Foundation, the nation's largest private philanthropy devoted to health care issues, was founded as a small local grantmaker in the mid-1930s by the late General Robert Wood Johnson, who built the Johnson & Johnson family of companies into a major international health and medical care products firm. A national foundation since 1972, it is a private, independent philanthropy unconnected to any corporate interests. More than $1 billion in grants have been awarded since 1972 to improve health care in the United States.

ISBN 0-942054-02-4

For additional free copies of this publication, write the address below or telephone 609/243-5934.

The Robert Wood Johnson Foundation
Post Office Box 2316
Princeton NJ 08543-2316

Table of Contents

INTRODUCTION

9 *Improving U.S. Health Care: An Overview of The Robert Wood Johnson Foundation's Grantmaking Program*
Leighton E. Cluff, MD

10 *An Overview of AIDS Programs Receiving Support from The Robert Wood Johnson Foundation*
Ruby P. Hearn, PhD

BACKGROUND ON THE STATUS OF THE AIDS EPIDEMIC

15 *Dispelling Myths About the AIDS Epidemic*
June E. Osborn, MD

22 *The AIDS Epidemic: Recent Trends and Future Prospects*
Jeffrey E. Harris, MD, PhD

29 □ Counterpoint   *Living With AIDS*
                        Buddy Clark

OVERVIEW OF THE CONTINUUM OF NEEDS AND RESPONSES BY COMMUNITIES

33 *The Robert Wood Johnson Foundation AIDS Prevention and Services Program: A Community Approach*
Edward N. Brandt, Jr., MD, PhD, and Deborah Lamm, MPA

36 □ Questions and Answers

37 *The Robert Wood Johnson Foundation AIDS Health Services Program*
Mervyn F. Silverman, MD, MPH

SPECIAL BURDENS ON INSTITUTIONS: RESULTS OF NEW STUDIES

45 *AIDS and HIV Treatment in our Cities' Public Hospitals, 1987-1988: Preliminary Analysis*
Dennis P. Andrulis, PhD

50 *The HIV-testing Policies of U.S. Hospitals*
Charles E. Lewis, MD, ScD, Kathleen Montgomery, PhD, and Christopher Corey, MA

54 □ Questions and Answers

TALE OF TWO CITIES: IN-DEPTH ANALYSIS OF RESPONSES TO THE CONTINUUM OF NEEDS

Dallas, Texas:
57 *Developing Coordinated Care for Persons With HIV Illness*
Warren W. Buckingham III

66 *The Evolution of an Epidemic: Parkland Memorial Hospital and the New Challenge of AIDS*
Ron J. Anderson, MD

Newark, New Jersey:

71   *Establishing an Integrated Network of AIDS Health Services*
     Steven R. Young, MSPH, and Adelaide Trautman, MD

76   □ Questions and Answers

AIDS Prevention for High-risk Populations

79   *The Chicago Adolescent AIDS Education Program*
     Douglas N. Bell

84   *The AIDS-HIV Prevention Program for Migrant Workers*
     Gail Anne Stevens

87   *The AIDS Prevention/Condom Promotion Project: Applying Effective Behavioral Change Techniques for Safer Sex*
     Deborah A. Cohen, MD

91   □ Questions and Answers

Community-based AIDS Support Services

95   *Project Open Hand: Home-delivered Meals for People With AIDS in San Francisco*
     Ruth Brinker

98   *Teleconference Education and Support Groups for People With AIDS in Rural Oklahoma*
     Marylee Behrens

101 *Assisting People With AIDS Through Volunteers of Legal Service, Inc.*
     William J. Dean

104 □ Questions and Answers

Housing and Long-term Care for People With AIDS

109 *AIDS: The Suburban Perspective*
     Gail Barouh, MA

116 *Providing Care in a County Nursing Home AIDS Unit*
     Shauna Dunn, RN, MS

120 *A Comprehensive Approach to AIDS Housing in a Second-Wave City: The Seattle-King County Model*
     Patricia L. McInturff, MPA

128 □ Questions and Answers

New Delivery and Payment Strategies: Some Options

133 *Human Immunodeficiency Virus Infection: Some Options for a Delivery and Payment Strategy*
     Donald A. Young, MD

141 *AIDS Prevention and Services: The Private Payer's Perspective*
     Carl J. Schramm, PhD, JD

144 *Putting AIDS Costs into Perspective: A Blue Cross and Blue Shield View*
Steven Sieverts

153 □ Questions and Answers

EDUCATION, TREATMENT, AND PAYMENT PRESSURES ON THE FEDERAL AND STATE GOVERNMENTS: PRESENTATIONS AND PANEL DISCUSSION

157 *Structural Barriers to Financing Early Intervention and Treatment for AIDS*
Timothy Westmoreland

161 *Problems in Administering the HRSA AIDS Programs: Short-term, Unpredictable and Rigid Funding Constraints*
Judith B. Braslow

163 *The Community Health Center Program*
Richard C. Bohrer

164 *Failures in Public Policy and the Crisis in HIV Care and Treatment in the United States, 1990*
Robert F. Hummel

167 *AIDS and the Medicaid Program: A View from the States*
Gary J. Clarke

171 *The Role of the States in Providing Financing and Access to HIV and AIDS Health Care Services*
Richard E. Merritt

175 □ Questions and Answers

181 *Closing Statement*
Paul S. Jellinek, PhD

AN OVERVIEW OF AIDS POLICY ISSUES

185 *Policy Considerations for AIDS: A Summary of Key Issues*
Deborah E. Lamm, MPA

INTRODUCTION

Improving U.S. Health Care: An Overview of The Robert Wood Johnson Foundation's Grantmaking Program

Leighton E. Cluff, MD

An Overview of AIDS Programs Receiving Support from The Robert Wood Johnson Foundation

Ruby P. Hearn, PhD

Improving U.S. Health Care: An Overview of The Robert Wood Johnson Foundation's Grantmaking Program

Leighton E. Cluff

The primary role of The Robert Wood Johnson Foundation, as one of the nation's largest private philanthropies, is to facilitate the work of others in improving health care for Americans. During its 18 years as a national foundation, it has awarded grants totaling over $1 billion. At present, the Foundation's grantmaking is focused on three broad areas: providing assistance to populations most vulnerable to illness, confronting the challenges posed by specific diseases of regional or national concern, and addressing a wide range of national health issues.

Foundation initiatives have included promoting the development of model health service projects, expanding health care and health policy research, and improving training for health professionals. Specific policy issues that have been explored with Foundation support include: the organization and financing of health services; quality of care; ethical issues in patient care; health care workforce concerns; and the impact of medical advances.

During the last five years, the Foundation has responded to a number of critical problems affecting high-risk groups in the U.S. population. To this end, the Foundation has made grants of more than $450 million to alleviate the problems of the homeless, the physically disabled, the elderly, those suffering from drug and alcohol abuse, adults and children with chronic mental illnesses, the uninsured, adolescents, and low birthweight, premature infants.

And, of course, people with AIDS. While clearly not an "AIDS foundation," The Robert Wood Johnson Foundation so far has been the principal source of private funds to provide preventive and health services for people with AIDS and HIV infection.

Looking toward the future, the Foundation plans to direct its grantmaking activities to other areas of need. Three new programs of special interest are: a program of community initiatives to reduce demand for illegal drugs and alcohol, a program to assist medical schools to prepare physicians better for the 21st century, and a program that helps hospitals strengthen patient care through institution-wide efforts to improve hospital nursing services.

America faces enormous challenges in meeting the current and future health care needs of our people. In particular, confronting the complex issues posed by the AIDS epidemic requires a nationwide commitment to action. My hope is that learning from one another—both service providers and policymakers—can be our next step toward achieving this commitment.

Leighton E. Cluff, MD, is the president of The Robert Wood Johnson Foundation (until July 1, 1990) and has served as a senior officer of the Foundation for 15 of its 18 years as a national philanthropy.

An Overview of AIDS Programs Receiving Support from The Robert Wood Johnson Foundation

Ruby P. Hearn

Introduction

The Robert Wood Johnson Foundation began its work in the AIDS area in 1985. Since that time it has provided over $50 million in support for more than 100 grants, well over half of all private philanthropic support devoted to AIDS. Our support has funded projects which have reached many thousands of people.

In 1985, Foundation staff began to explore the emerging AIDS epidemic to determine whether there was a possible role for the Foundation. For several reasons, we weren't sure there was. At that time, the major challenges appeared to be in the areas of biomedical research, epidemiologic research, and public education. We believed that biomedical and epidemiologic research were the provinces of the federal government, and—at that time—public education was not a priority for the Foundation. As you may recall, there also was considerable controversy as to just what educational messages should be conveyed to the general public. Furthermore, the Foundation's expertise in grantmaking had been in the area of the delivery of health services, especially out-of-hospital care.

The breakthrough for us came with the identification of San Francisco's Comprehensive AIDS Service Program, which provided a model that responded to certain important facts about AIDS. Despite the high fatality rate and short life expectancy for AIDS patients, it was already becoming clear that people with AIDS required extensive medical and support services outside the hospital. Hospitals were feeling the strain from the lack of out-of-hospital placement options for AIDS patients, and San Francisco had begun to address this problem. They had developed an innovative system of community-based services for patients with AIDS that had reduced the need for prolonged and repeated hospitalizations.

Community-based Services

After visiting San Francisco, the staff concluded that an important Foundation contribution would be to help other communities develop similar community-based systems of care for AIDS patients. In 1985 we made our first grant in the AIDS area to the AIDS Health Policy Institute at the University of California at San Francisco, to support the dissemination of information to clinicians, policymakers and other groups about San Francisco's program. At the same time, the Foundation's Board of Trustees authorized the AIDS Health Services Program, a $17.2 million national demonstration program. Its goals are to stimulate the development of community-based services for people with HIV infection in 11 communities around the country and to test the viability of this approach in very diverse settings—Atlanta, Dallas, Fort Lauderdale, Jersey City, Miami, Nassau County (NY), Newark (NJ), New Orleans, New York City, Seattle, and West Palm Beach. The Foundation is also currently funding an independent evaluation by Brown University, which is studying changes in service utilization patterns, the quality of patient care services, and the implementation process for the 11 community projects.

Ruby P. Hearn, PhD, is a vice president of The Robert Wood Johnson Foundation.

AIDS Prevention Education

In the fall of 1986, two major AIDS reports were issued—one by former Surgeon General C. Everett Koop and the other by the National Academy of Sciences' Institutes of Medicine. Both called for major national efforts in AIDS prevention education. With no vaccine or cure on the horizon, the only strategy that appeared feasible to slow the spread of the epidemic was prevention of HIV infection. During an extensive review of possible strategies for the Foundation in the prevention area and an analysis of current funding patterns in both the public and private sectors, the staff concluded that a large number of community groups and local organizations were poised to provide preventive services but were having great difficulty in securing funding.

Therefore, in March 1988, we issued a call for proposals to support AIDS prevention and service projects focusing on those groups at greatest risk for the disease. This call for proposals was unprecedented for the Foundation, in that it specified no predetermined level of funding for either individual grants or the total program. We wanted to reach out to agencies and organizations that had no previous contact with the Foundation, and we cast a wide net in search of innovative approaches.

By the July 1988 deadline, we had received more than 1,000 proposals requesting over $500 million. They came from almost every state and territory. Over half came from community organizations, and individual requests ranged from $1,000 to $10 million. After an extensive multi-phase review, we selected 54 projects, totaling almost $17 million, to be recommended to the Foundation's Trustees for support. These projects have just completed their first year of implementation. They already are demonstrating the potential for organizations and groups of all kinds—not only health care providers, but also church groups, schools, labor unions, PTAs, Girls Clubs, and law firms—to play a direct and meaningful role in helping their communities respond to AIDS.

This overwhelming response to the call for proposals was an important measure of the growing level of concern and readiness to confront the epidemic at the community level. The Foundation issued a memorandum detailing this to 900 legislators, governors, mayors, federal agencies, and leaders in the private and voluntary sectors.

Research and Policy Efforts

In addition to our support for these two national programs, the Foundation has supported a number of single-grant projects to generate and disseminate information about the epidemic and its impact. These include:

☐ annual surveys about the impact of AIDS on the nation's hospitals (The potential impact of the epidemic on hospitals had been an important consideration in the Foundation's decision to launch the AIDS Health Services Program and was of growing concern to administrators and policymakers.)

☐ a nationwide survey of hospital AIDS testing policies and practices

☐ the development of a dynamic simulation model for forecasting the incidence and case-mix of the epidemic into the late 1990s, taking into account various alternative scenarios regarding the development of preventive and treatment interventions

☐ establishment of the New York-New Jersey Citizens Commission on AIDS and shortly thereafter the National Leadership Coalition on AIDS, both of which seek to engage the business and voluntary sectors in improving public understanding of the issues surrounding AIDS and improving the coordination of public and private sector activities, and

☐ the establishment of a state AIDS policy center to provide timely and objective AIDS policy information to state, county, and local officials across the country.

Recognizing that public policy is very much influenced by the general public's attitudes and concerns regarding a problem, we identified another role for the Foundation: to make available balanced, objective information about the epidemic and its impact on families and institutions in a readily accessible format. We were concerned that the public was dependent on episodic, often sensational reporting and that there was no ongoing effort to provide accurate and timely information. Thus, in 1988, the Foundation provided a $4 million grant to WGBH in Boston to enable the producers of *Nova* and *Frontline* to develop *The AIDS Quarterly* for broadcast on public television. The Foundation recently renewed its support to WGBH for two additional episodes in 1990.

Financing Issues

From our experience to date, many communities clearly are mobilizing to respond to the AIDS epidemic. Furthermore, we have seen that the community-based systems approach does work: Case management can be implemented even in the most varied and difficult environments, as you will hear later from the AIDS Health Services Program projects.

The major challenge is, of course, financing. The feasibility of delivering a continuum of community-based services has been demonstrated—both in Foundation-supported programs and in projects funded by the federal government—but unless there are major changes in financing, this concept will not flourish and will not be replicated in the many other communities where it is needed.

The Foundation's projects are now trying to patch together a variety of funding sources to keep their activities going. We continue to monitor the situation, both in terms of the status of the epidemic and in terms of the federal, state, and private sector responses. And, we will continue to assess whether there is anything further that the Foundation can do to help the country confront this epidemic.

But, as you know, philanthropic support alone cannot hope to meet more than a fraction of the total need for services and education in any major health area, including AIDS. The Foundation's most important role, as we see it, is to test new approaches to addressing major health problems and to learn what works and what doesn't, in the hope that this information will be of value to those who have the responsibility for policymaking and service delivery.

The purpose of this conference is to provide an opportunity for some of the Foundation's AIDS grantees to share with you what they are learning. To provide a context for our workshop, June Osborn will discuss some of the myths about the AIDS epidemic, and Jeffrey Harris will provide an overview of how the epidemic is likely to unfold in the 1990s.

Then, we will move on to a review of specific projects that are trying to address some of the most difficult problems, including the development of a continuum of care in the community, preventing the spread of the epidemic to those at highest risk, and the provision of support services, housing, and long-term care. We will conclude the meeting with what we hope will be a productive discussion of how to pay for all of these much-needed services.

BACKGROUND ON THE STATUS OF THE AIDS EPIDEMIC

Dispelling Myths About the AIDS Epidemic
June E. Osborn, MD

The AIDS Epidemic: Recent Trends and Future Prospects
Jeffrey E. Harris, MD, PhD

☐ Counterpoint   *Living With AIDS*
                     Buddy Clark

DISPELLING MYTHS ABOUT THE AIDS EPIDEMIC

June E. Osborn

(from a presentation given to the Economic Club of Grand Rapids [MI] on February 5, 1990, and adapted for the AIDS Prevention and Services Workshop)

It must be difficult in this country for a thoughtful person to make sense out of the mixed messages about AIDS. As an example, concerned medical and political leaders persist in urgent efforts to attract public attention to a real and expanding disaster, and yet nowhere was the AIDS epidemic addressed in the 1990 State of the Union message—nor has it ever been, despite the fact that the numbers of Americans caught up in this horror have escalated more and more dramatically over the past decade.

More than 120,000 Americans have been diagnosed with AIDS during that time, and nearly 70,000 of them have died. Even the most conservative estimates suggest that these numbers will more than double in the next two years, that now nearly 1,000,000 Americans face future premature illness from HIV infection and that the minimum number of new infections each year is 45,000, with the more likely number two to five times that—90,000 to 225,000. Since the average interval between onset of infection with the human immunodeficiency virus (or HIV) and onset of AIDS is at least 10 years, each increment assures us of AIDS trouble further into the 21st century.

Americans are, under most circumstances, a strikingly compassionate people. Think, for instance, of the little Texas girl who fell into a well—or of the outpouring of concern for the youngster who was the sole survivor of an airplane crash in Detroit a couple of years ago. One would have thought that such terrible numbers of sick young adults facing personal tragedy would have us all scrambling to plan for the care of the sick, to double-check and reinforce the efficacy of our educational weapons to protect our children, and to assist those already infected to gain access to new delaying therapies that might buy precious time for more biomedical progress.

And yet it isn't working like that. AIDS has dropped off the media screen for the most part, and when it appears it takes confusingly mixed forms of upbeat coverage about vaccine progress, revisions of projections from one six-digit number to another, or even snarling accusations that it was all a great hoax. Only occasionally are there somber and complex pieces such as Peter Jennings's *The AIDS Quarterly* that can be found on PBS, and they probably mean most to the already-converted.

You may be under the impression that at least public education is going well, yet in many parts of the U.S. the public service announcements are solely those sanitized messages from the federal government, shown "after the late, late show and before the sermonette," as Dr. Mervyn Silverman likes to point out.

Worse than mixed messages and half-hearted efforts at education, however, is the new spate of articles and op-ed pieces suggesting that we AIDS folks are somehow misleading the public. Either our motives are questioned or we are dubbed the "AIDS establishment," suggesting a power that leaves me wishing I knew how to find it and exercise it—because there really is big trouble already, and much worse is guaranteed to come before things let up! Just for the record, let me assure you: I do not have nefarious

June E. Osborn, MD, chairs the National Commission on AIDS. Since 1984, she has been the dean of the School of Public Health at the University of Michigan. She also chairs The Robert Wood Johnson Foundation's National Advisory Committee for the AIDS Health Services Program.

agendas beyond caring greatly about America and about the health of the public, and I did not make up the depressing things I need to talk to you about!

Now that the federal budget season is upon us, the cumulative effect of this cacophony is downright scary, for out of the mix of messages have come some myths that one really wants to believe, for instance: "It isn't going to be as bad as they said, is it?" or "Now that there is something we can do for those people, they should all be tested" or "Heterosexual AIDS doesn't really happen—it's just those drug addicts." The ultimate anxiety-reliever, I think, is the business about a vaccine, something like: "I hear they've made progress with a vaccine, so it should be over soon, right?" Wrong. But we'll get to that in due course.

In this presentation I will address these specific sources of confusion, for it is most important that we see our problem with HIV and AIDS quite clearly. The virus of AIDS is a sexually transmitted pathogen, and while it varies in efficiency depending on specific kinds of sexual activity, any variety of sexual intercourse works. Birth to an infected mother or injection of substantial quantities of blood through transfusion or drug use are the only alternative modes of spread. That means that knowledge about sexual and drug-associated risk empowers people to decide on a personal policy of avoidance, and of course it also means that ignorance can be disastrous.

Jim Curran of the CDC used to say in the epidemic's early years that in 1990 people would be shaking their fists at us saying "Why didn't you tell us?" Well, 1990 is here now, and were not so many people grieving in secret for fear of disgrace or discrimination, we would already know how vast the problem is. I suspect—in view of the sheer numbers of AIDS diagnoses being made—that by the end of the year, Jim's prediction will have come to pass, and we will look back in shame as a society for having failed to take advantage of our knowledge. For that reason if no other, AIDS must concern us all.

I should probably tell you right away why I say that AIDS is everyone's problem, for I realize that in many people the response is "Not me!" One day I was doing a C-SPAN talk show and made that statement—about our need as a human family to recognize the universality of risk. A man called in and took me to task, saying that he had been happily and monogamously married for 25 years and did not think he was at risk. I told him that I agreed with him in the narrow sense and apologized for seeming to overstate my case; but then I pointed out that what he said about himself might not pertain to his children, or to his children's children. Few of us can be sure that we know everything about our children—in Khalil Gibran's beautiful book, one of my favorite passages is the Prophet's powerful admonition about children: "They dwell in the house of tomorrow where you may never enter." In that sense it is absolutely critical that we recognize that, like the day after Hiroshima, the world has changed and will never be the same again. The virus of AIDS is a new and permanent menace; it is "out there" to threaten, but we are not powerless if we take pains to teach our children frankly and forthrightly to avoid it.

The "Not-So-Bad" Myth of AIDS—Confusion about the Data

Let's look at the "AIDS is not-so-bad" myth first. This myth comes partly from genuine disagreements among experts concerning projections. It also comes from appropriate revisions of earlier estimates in the face of new knowledge. Please bear with us for that—the epidemic is less than 10 years old in its recognized form, the virus was only discovered in 1983, and we have had to learn as we coped with a burgeoning public health disaster. If the U.S. Public Health Service is better now than in 1986 at assessing trends and projecting, it is a testimony to progress, not a demonstration of prior ineptitude.

In terms of total numbers infected, one cannot be precise, but even the smallest number suggested for

16

Americans infected as of 1986—in light of all the new data and improvements—is 600,000. New infections will have brought that by now to at least 1,000,000 by almost everyone's assessment. That's awful! What is this business about "just" 600,000? Remember how upset we were about 221 cases of Legionnaire's Disease in 1976?

As to cases of AIDS, we know unequivocally that 120,000 have been diagnosed thus far and that about 70,000 have died. Here comes a point of genuinely confusing data, however, for there seems to have been a slowing down of diagnosed AIDS cases around 1987. What is that about? In the answer lies the main thrust of my message, and it has great bearing as well on the second myth I mentioned—that we should now test everybody since there is so much that can (theoretically) be done for them. I know in detail about these data, because I reviewed the manuscript in which they were presented in order to write an accompanying editorial.

First, what do these numbers say? The authors carefully analyzed the turndown in reported AIDS cases and looked at whether it was uniform—they found that it was not. Rather, it was seen in those relatively affluent, educated populations where both awareness of and access to progress in clinical care was most likely; however, it was not seen in the growing fraction of the population at high risk from circumstances where poverty, relative illiteracy and absence of health care options are the rule. For this and other reasons, they concluded persuasively that the turndown was testimony to the progress that has been made in clinical approaches and treatment of persons with AIDS.

However, several caveats were important. The most somber of these was that their entire analysis dealt with AIDS as a formal diagnostic category, not with the full spectrum of HIV disease. It is important to emphasize that AIDS is the finale in a progressive process of immunologic deficit mediated by the virus and that treatments available may delay but do not cure the underlying problem or permanently interrupt the progression. It is almost certain that the turndown represents a slowing of the onset of AIDS; but remember, those infected people are still there, still infected, and we are sadly certain they will become ill later. We have simply bought some time and postponed the inevitable.

Factors in the Turndown in AIDS Cases

Still, it is worth a moment to celebrate progress. At present it is generally agreed that a cure for AIDS is not around the corner. Instead, the clinician's goal is to turn HIV disease into a chronic, livable condition analogous to diabetes—in other words, to delay AIDS as long as possible—and the news is that we have made measurable progress toward that achievable goal.

Pneumocystis carinii pneumonia is the biggest single killer of persons with AIDS as well as being the most common infection that allows physicians to make the diagnosis. The capacity of nebulized therapy to stave it off or prevent recurrences when administered monthly surely has contributed to delaying AIDS diagnoses—but wait and look. The drug for this (called pentamidine) is expensive, nebulizers are scarce, and to take advantage of this intervention, one needs to have a usable relationship with a physician or at least with a responsive health care system. All these prerequisites to appropriate care have become a sad new kind of definition of affluence in America. The poor cannot even find primary care, much less take advantage of this elegant realization of our biomedical progress.

As you have read, there is a drug called AZT (or sometimes zidovudine) that works directly against the virus of AIDS and has been shown to buy precious months for people with AIDS during which they feel better and sometimes even return to work and normal functioning. It doesn't last indefinitely, sadly, and it has serious toxicity problems, but it does offer real time and invaluable hope. Recently it has been found that by giving it earlier, before HIV disease has progressed to the AIDS diagnosis, one can do even better and with lower doses, which help to decrease the toxic effects a great deal.

Even though the drug has been around for only a couple of years, there is already persuasive evidence that it has played a role in the slowdown of progression to AIDS. But AZT is an even more dramatically uneven health care option than is pentamidine, for it is ferociously expensive (not as expensive, I should note, as even a few days in the hospital—but third-party payors are used to paying for hospitalization, and outpatient therapy with AZT has presented new issues).

At several thousand dollars a year, middle-income people have been brought to their financial knees by the burden of AZT's cost. Even the well-insured and the very affluent are stunned. Inclusion of AZT as a Medicaid option has been met by a number of states with reluctance or, horribly, with refusal until lately. As recently as July of 1989 there were still two states in this wealthy land where AZT simply was not available if one was poor. For the rest, Congress provided uneasy respite (albeit grudgingly) with six-month extensions of federal support for this life-sustaining option via Medicaid. It is my information that it is once again missing from the President's budget, as is financing of home care. The latter could help to reduce the burden on the tertiary care hospitals that are figuratively collapsing and literally closing their doors in some cities that are epicenters of the epidemic.

Besides these two costly but effective pharmacologic interventions that clearly can delay the diagnosis of AIDS, it has become evident that the heroic physicians who have cared for burgeoning numbers of persons with AIDS have been learning in the midst of crisis. It has been increasingly evident that comprehensive clinical care can add significantly to both the number and the quality of months remaining to persons with HIV disease. While some "underground" efforts in this respect have led to exotic diets, supplements and regimens of unlikely value, there is now good reason to conclude that careful maintenance of nutrition is a powerful adjunct to specific therapies and that the dreadful wasting that is part of the virus's effect can play a primary or determinant role in the rate of disease progression.

It stands to reason that early treatment to decrease the pain of oral thrush or herpes, to deal with symptomatic dental decay and to combat the awful synergy of HIV and lack of appetite all enhance the likelihood of sustained survival. I have suspected for many years that those AIDS clinicians were true heros; now one can see validation of their feats even in the relatively insensitive measures of population-based statistics.

Before the celebration gets out of hand, however, it must be noted that some other factors could be contributing to the downturn in numbers of AIDS diagnoses. Underreporting is always a problem in keeping data of this kind, but in a dreadfully stigmatizing disease, underreporting may be distributed unevenly. A caring physician may find it easiest to diagnose pneumonia or cancer and leave the rest unspoken, especially if the community response to full medical disclosure is likely to be devastating to survivors.

Bisexuality is an important part of this epidemic, and as the term suggests, a grieving wife and children may be at risk of post-mortem outrage if AIDS is clearly identified. Many physicians have told me privately that this concern enters their thinking about reporting, filling out death certificates and the like. It is impossible to know how large an effect this could have on the apparent reporting "deficit," but it is certain that it would be greater in that part of our population privileged to enjoy compassionate, personalized care.

Even the less advantaged may be diagnosed less often than they might be, for a very different reason—which is that they die before they qualify for formal "AIDS" diagnosis. Among drug users, for instance, there has always been a propensity to serious infections; it has now been clearly shown that some of those infections may be taking on added virulence in the presence of underlying HIV and carrying people off before they ever have time to progress to AIDS itself. Clearly this represents another source of artifactual data, if one uses AIDS (rather than HIV disease) as a barometer of epidemic pressure. Undercounting the "underclass" cases of HIV-related mortality occurs for very different reasons, but again the number of AIDS cases is lower as a result, and the human cost of the HIV epidemic is further underassessed.

So the statements that "It is not so bad," that "The numbers are smaller than we thought," that "Now that there is something we can do everyone should come forward"—all these myths are sprinkled with bits of fact, but they don't play straightforwardly. More accurately, the numbers are dreadful, access to health care is cruelly uneven, and to urge that people be tested when discrimination is out there and treatment isn't is rather grotesque.

Heterosexual AIDS—Not a Myth

But we AIDS Establishment people are also accused of spreading myths, such as the "myth of heterosexual AIDS." Some of you may have seen the book of that name that was just published, and while its author deserves a hearing and is technically correct in saying that the proportion of purely heterosexually spread cases has remained fairly steady in the U.S., the very title of the book renders an awful disservice.

Heterosexual AIDS is no myth. There have been more cases of heterosexual AIDS in the U.S. thus far than most other countries have in total cases of any sort—and the recorded history of the epidemic is not yet a decade old! From earliest times, it was clear that heterosexual partners of persons infected with HIV were themselves at risk. In large parts of the world, HIV is predominantly a heterosexually spread disease, and we Americans are not a different species. If one watches U.S. trends, women are the fastest growing component of the epidemic; male-to-female ratios of infected people have been dropping steadily so that they are 3:1 in numerous national surveys (compared to 11:1 years ago) and are nearing 1:1 in areas where the virus has been around the longest. Should we be comfortable about that? As I noted earlier, what is at issue here is the efficiency of sexual spread, not its occurrence!

A Vaccine for AIDS—Not a Panacea

Finally, progress with a vaccine—what about it? I confess this distractor makes me a bit tired, for I am a veteran of old vaccine wars and believe me, a perfect vaccine ready at hand would not do much for us at our present juncture. It would be a great help in countries where the nearly complete lack of health care infrastructure makes AIDS a cataclysmic "last straw," but in the U.S., we should not even be tempted to temporize or wait. The fact is that a vaccine for widespread use against AIDS is a long way off, despite intermittent excitement in the press. It is relatively little the fault of the scientists involved in the important search for a future vaccine strategy that every technological tidbit or twitch commands such brassy media attention; but we should know from past experience that vaccines are not panaceas.

The "vaccine-is-near" myth has serious consequences, though, for it excuses people from paying attention to tough messages about behavior modification. It is a happy fact that, with secure blood screening policies and procedures in place as they are now, this virus can be avoided by personal decision-making about behavior, and there will never be a vaccine as good as that. Education has been aptly referred to as the vaccine against HIV. But of course, just as a vaccine is of no use in its bottle, so education for prevention is of no use if not delivered diligently, clearly, and in the language of the intended listener.

AIDS Not Under Control

There is one other common perception I didn't get to, but given that it is the budget time of year, perhaps I should. Increasingly one hears that "AIDS is just one disease, and we've put a lot of resources into it—now we have to back off, to be fair to other diseases." To this one I say that the only new thing about AIDS is the virus itself. Almost all of the problems we are faced with in health care, its financing, and the like are old ones that have been patched over or ignored; and the effort we devote to their solution will have benefits far beyond the scope of AIDS. In particular, as I said earlier, it is increasingly becoming a chronic, treatable disease, and our urgent need to innovate options to provide for a continuum of care raises many of the issues that our elderly could have told us about long ago. If we meet the challenge thoughtfully, our efforts can have positive impact far beyond the immediate crisis of the HIV epidemic.

Furthermore, I think on the research side that the insights accruing in many areas of so-called AIDS research will have a rich harvest leading to progress in many other areas—most notably cancer, progressive neurologic disorders, and some of the chronic arthritides.

One other comment about the "just-one-disease" myth: AIDS is a disease unlike any other competing for attention, in that it is communicable, the numbers are not static and indeed are escalating rapidly, it has a long silent interval prior to its inexorable expression, and the fact that it is preventable means that further spread is unconscionable. In those senses, unlike other diseases, it is not yet anywhere near control—and that is very different from other diseases.

I am by nature a very hopeful, upbeat person, but in my role as chairwoman of the National Commission on AIDS I often feel that I must play the role of Cassandra, and this is one of those times. If I were to join in celebration of incremental progress, there would be a great risk of misinterpretation. There is such a long way yet to go. A sense that the end is in sight might let health care workers continue to indulge in the fantasy that they can avoid working with HIV-infected people (in their minds they say "AIDS patients" which is how the fantasy survives). Communities, and for that matter Congress, could continue to opine that "We've done enough for AIDS," just as the tidal wave of health care need approaches their shores. And people could continue to take false solace from titles such as *The Myth of Heterosexual AIDS* while 10-year ticking time bombs are planted unnoticed among their sexually active children.

So I must persevere as Cassandra: The broad outlines of the next decade's stressful times have been defined for us, and were there not another single instance of transmission of HIV, we would have overwhelming trouble ahead. Even with the progress that has slowed the advent of AIDS as a final diagnosis, enormous numbers of Americans are "in the pipeline" and will soon require our help to live out their truncated lives with productivity while possible, with access to health care as needed, and with dignity throughout.

I have a favorite joke about the airline pilot who comes on the PA system and says, "Well folks, there's good news and there's bad news. The good news is that we're making great time. The bad news is, we're lost." Indeed, in historical perspective, we—especially the scientists and clinicians—are making great time. The awful bad news is that as a society responding to AIDS as an historic challenge, Americans may be getting lost. We must stop arguing among ourselves whether 600,000 or 900,000 is a large number, or whether we can afford to devote one or two percent of our total health care expenditures to deal with a crippling and ultimately lethal disease that is devouring our youth.

We need instead to recognize that the biomedical progress to date has bought us precious time to make desperately needed adjustments in our health care system. We need revision of health care financing, creation of outpatient and home care options, training of case managers to guide sick people through the health care maze, and extensive education of health care professionals so that the fruits of that progress may be accessible more and more broadly.

I don't want to dilute my earlier theme of HIV as a universal risk too much, for that is the AIDS message I most want you to retain. But beyond the accumulating personal tragedies and behind the grieving-in-secret lies a societal matter that should concern us all, as well. To illustrate my thought, let me take a brief diversion to a related topic.

One Human Family in Fighting AIDS

A thoughtful editorial about homelessness recently in the *Journal of the American Medical Association* included a quotation by an American poet of an earlier era talking about war—I don't know which war, but I suspect it might well have been the First World War. The quotation is: "The most tragic thing about the war was not that it made so many dead men, but that it destroyed the tragedy of death." The author added his observation that "the greatest loss of the 1980s is that American homelessness and poverty are no longer tragedies but the acceptable cost of our affluence."

I would like to add to that thinking that the face of a potential tragedy of the 1990s is becoming ever more clear, for we are toying openly with the rationalization that AIDS is a disease of "them, not us," and that we have done more than enough about it already, since it is happening to "others." Even as we have made progress, there are now data to prove that as of 1987, when it came to AIDS, it mattered more than ever who you were, who you knew, and what you earned.

Numerically, the HIV epidemic in the decade of the 1990s will be far worse than what we have seen so far, and it will touch us all. We must not tolerate the perpetuation of that immoral distortion of a society dedicated to the importance of each individual life. Remember, we are all part of one human family—there are no "others!"

THE AIDS EPIDEMIC:
RECENT TRENDS AND FUTURE PROSPECTS

Jeffrey E. Harris

The Deceleration in AIDS Incidence

Recent evidence suggests a possible slowdown in the growth rate of new AIDS cases (see Figure 1). The apparent slowing in overall AIDS incidence has occurred predominantly among homosexual and bisexual men, who still make up most of the cases (see Figure 2).[1] This slowdown in AIDS diagnoses among homosexual men has been observed primarily in San Francisco, New York and Los Angeles, but also among white men outside these major coastal cities.[2]

There are three competing, but not mutually exclusive, explanations for the observed slowdown in AIDS incidence. First, the trend may be an artifact of increasing underreporting of AIDS cases over the past two years. Second, zidovudine (AZT) and aerosolized pentamidine may have been administered to growing numbers of HIV-infected patients before they manifested AIDS.[3] Third, the slowdown could be the

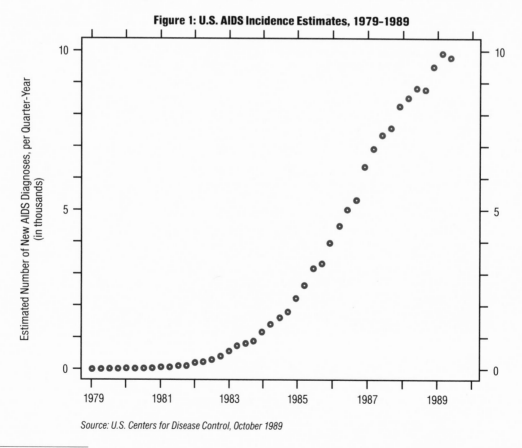

Figure 1: U.S. AIDS Incidence Estimates, 1979–1989

Estimated Number of New AIDS Diagnoses, per Quarter-Year (in thousands)

Source: U.S. Centers for Disease Control, October 1989

Jeffrey E. Harris, MD, PhD, serves as economics professor at the Massachusetts Institute of Technology, where he teaches health economics and statistics. He is also an internist at Boston's Massachusetts General Hospital, where his medical practice includes people with HIV infection.

consequence of a decline in the incidence of HIV infection several years earlier.

It is not possible with current data to distinguish sharply among these three competing explanations. An increase in the underreporting of AIDS is not likely to be the sole explanation. Although certain manifestations of AIDS are known to be seriously underreported among intravenous drug users,[4] the apparent slowdown in AIDS incidence has occurred not in that group but among white homosexual men. Still, AIDS has probably been diagnosed increasingly on an outpatient basis, as patients have sought medical care earlier in the course of their disease. It is possible that state and local health departments have been less successful in identifying such outpatient cases.

Zidovudine has been available in the United States since late 1986. At about the same time, oral trimethoprim-sulfamethoxazole and aerosolized pentamidine began to be used to prevent *Pneumocystis carinii* pneumonia (PCP). Both treatments have now entered into widespread clinical use, at least for patients with confirmed AIDS. Clinical trials have confirmed that zidovudine delays the progression to AIDS in asymptomatic HIV-infected patients with severe immune deficiency (defined as fewer than 500 CD4+ cells per cubic millimeter).[5] The critical unanswered question, however, is how many such HIV-infected patients received treatment during the past two or three years?

Based upon unit sales of zidovudine, an estimated 40,000 to 80,000 patients are currently taking the drug in the United States. About 4,000 eligible patients with AIDS took advantage of the zidovudine compassionate plea program during late 1986 and early 1987.[6] For the sake of argument, suppose that 5,000 asymptomatic HIV-infected patients with depressed immune systems (CD4+ counts under 500) had been taking zidovudine during 1987, and that 10,000 were taking the drug in 1988. For such patients,

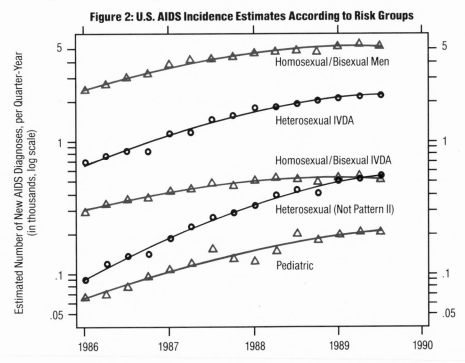

Figure 2: U.S. AIDS Incidence Estimates According to Risk Groups

NOTES: "IVDA" means intravenous drug abuser. "Pediatric" means AIDS patients under age 13 at the time of diagnosis. "Heterosexual (Not Pattern II)" means heterosexual AIDS patients who were not born in those countries (especially in Africa) where heterosexual transmission of human immunodeficiency virus (HIV) is prevalent, in order to exclude AIDS patients who probably acquired their HIV infections outside the United States.

zidovudine reduces the one-year rate of progression to AIDS five percent to two percent, and the two-year rate of progression is reduced from 15 percent to eight percent.[7] At best, only about 700 or 800 cases of AIDS would have been prevented by such treatment.

In order to explore the third explanation for the slowed AIDS rate—that there was an earlier decline in HIV infection—a simple "back calculation" model of HIV incidence may be used.[8] The idea behind such a model is to reconstruct the number of past cases of HIV infection that would be required to produce the current pattern of new AIDS cases. Making such a calculation requires information on the incubation period of HIV.[9]

Figure 3 repeats CDC's data on actual AIDS incidence from Figure 1 and shows two estimates of AIDS incidence derived from different back calculation models.[10] Model A's estimates were based upon all of the AIDS incidence data from the first quarter of 1979 through the third quarter of 1989. In Model B, the same statistical procedure was employed, but the last six data-points were dropped, so that only the incidence data through the first quarter of 1988 were included. For both models, the fitted incidence of AIDS is also projected forward through 1992.

Published projections of future AIDS cases have changed considerably over the past few years.[11] Comparison of these projections is difficult, because both the projection models and the underlying data have changed. The analysis in Figure 3, by contrast, applies the same statistical model to two different data bases. This figure shows how strongly updated AIDS incidence data influence future AIDS projections.

The differences between Models A and B are substantial. An analyst who used only the AIDS incidence data available as of early 1988 (Model B) would project 142,000 AIDS cases by the third quarter of 1989—

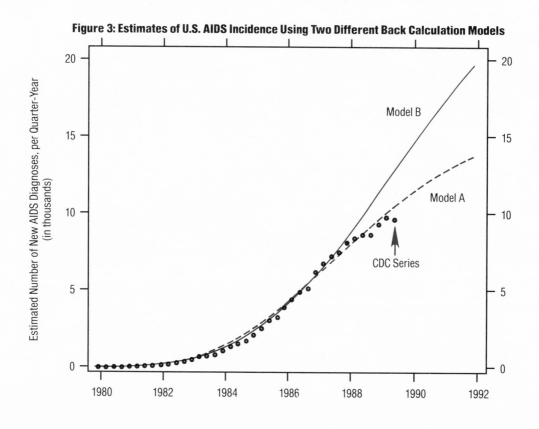

Figure 3: Estimates of U.S. AIDS Incidence Using Two Different Back Calculation Models

about 11,000 cases more than are currently estimated by the CDC. The same analyst would project a cumulative total of 680,000 AIDS cases by 1996—about 198,000 more than are projected by Model A.

A more detailed look at Model A is shown in Figure 4, which plots the estimated incidence of HIV infection since 1977. Also plotted are CDC's actual AIDS incidence data and the AIDS incidence projected through 1995. According to Model A, HIV infections peaked in 1983 at about 53,000 cases per quarter-year (95 percent confidence interval, ±2,000) and fell markedly by 1985 to about 12,000 (95 percent confidence interval, ±2,000). A continued linear decline in new HIV infections since 1985 would produce an estimated 6,800 new HIV cases per quarter-year in mid-1989. Moreover, the predicted future incidence of AIDS reaches a relatively flat maximum in the range of 14,000 new cases per quarter-year during 1992-1996.

By contrast, Model B does not produce a downturn in new HIV infections after 1983. The estimated HIV incidence, in fact, increases from 39,000 in 1983 (95 percent confidence interval, ±3,000) to 41,000 in 1985 (95 percent confidence interval, ±2,000). Even if HIV incidence declined linearly thereafter, the estimated HIV incidence would be 23,500 cases per quarter-year in mid-1989.

Both Model A and Model B were applied to CDC's AIDS incidence data that are uncorrected for underreporting of AIDS cases.[12] If the extent of underreporting has been 20 percent over the course of the epidemic, then the estimates all need to be adjusted upward by a factor of 1.25. Still, comparison of the models suggests that the recent AIDS incidence falls short of that which could have been predicted in early 1988 by at least 11,000 cases. Moreover, the slowdown is consistent with a downturn in HIV infections after 1983.

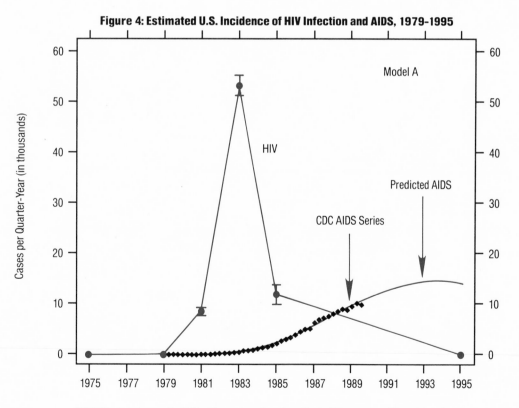

Figure 4: Estimated U.S. Incidence of HIV Infection and AIDS, 1979-1995

NOTE: The error bars on the HIV incidence curve show the estimated 95 percent confidence intervals.

25

Seroprevalence data from selected cohorts of homosexual men suggest that the incidence of new HIV infections was declining after 1982.[13] However, these cohorts are small. Taken together, they contain only about 5,000 subjects who were initially seronegative, and there is no guarantee that these cohorts are representative of HIV infection among homosexual men generally. Although there is evidence that sexual practices among homosexual men were changing as early as 1982,[14] even without such behavioral change, HIV infection rates could still decline, as the very highest risk groups of homosexual men became almost fully infected.[15]

If the recent slowdown in AIDS cases is a real consequence of an earlier peaking in HIV incidence, can we be confident that it is permanent? Figure 2 shows that heterosexual AIDS cases continue to increase among both intravenous drug users and their heterosexual partners. While AIDS incidence in these groups is still a minority of all cases, this situation may change in the late 1990s.

The Improvement in Survival of AIDS Patients

Recent studies[16] have shown a trend toward improved short-term survival from AIDS, at least since 1986. The gain in survival, however, has been seen only in AIDS patients initially manifesting PCP.[17] The reduced mortality among PCP patients was seen in every risk group. Among homosexual men the increase in median survival for PCP patients was particularly pronounced, increasing from 10.5 months in 1984 to 18.0 months in 1987.

The apparent improvement in survival could conceivably be due to the growing difficulties in ascertaining AIDS-related mortality. Even in a carefully followed cohort of AIDS patients in San Francisco, mortality status could not be determined in 10 percent of cases.[18] But it is hardly clear how such a bias in mortality follow-up would be confined to PCP patients in every risk group. Alternatively, the apparent gain in survival could be the consequence of earlier diagnosis of AIDS, when patients are at a less advanced stage of HIV infection; however, this hypothesis is weakened by the fact that very little of the mortality decline was observed immediately after diagnosis. The observed improvements in survival in the 1986 and 1987 cohorts are most consistent with the introduction of new medical therapies in 1986 and 1987. Zidovudine, in particular, was approved by the U.S. Food and Drug Administration in 1987 for use in AIDS patients with a confirmed episode of PCP.

Will the initial decline in mortality continue? If so, what will the prevalence of AIDS be as we approach the mid-1990s? Preliminary data from 1988 and 1989 do indeed suggest a continued mortality decline, but these improvements continue to be confined to PCP patients. If the gain in survival actually reflects the increased use of zidovudine, and if the drug is also effective in AIDS patients without PCP, then future gains in survival for non-PCP patients are possible. Whether zidovudine will improve long-term survival and whether other antiviral agents will soon enter widespread clinical use are questions critical to any future mortality projections.

To gain some understanding of the potential impact of future improvements in survival, I used the estimates from Models A and B to project AIDS incidence and prevalence through the first quarter of 1996. My key assumption was that median survival progressively increased from about 15 months in 1987 to 30 months by 1996. If so, the great majority of patients who contracted AIDS during 1976-1996 will be alive in 1996. Under Model A, about 482,000 AIDS cases will have occurred by 1996, of which about 315,000 will still be alive.

What will be the impact of over 300,000 people living with AIDS? That is about one AIDS patient for every three acute care hospital beds in the United States. But the issue for the medical care system—and for our economy generally—is really the health status of AIDS patients and not merely their number. If antiviral therapy decreases the frequency and severity of AIDS-associated opportunistic infections, then conceivably many AIDS patients will remain out of the hospital and in the workplace.

Model A gives a cumulative incidence of HIV infection of nearly 780,000 cases by 1996. A reasonable correction for underreporting of AIDS cases would boost the HIV infection estimate to about one million. If HIV infection rates continue to decline, then about 60 percent of the cumulative total of HIV-infected persons will have already contracted AIDS by 1996, and the remaining 40 percent will be in various pre-AIDS stages in the natural history of HIV infection. Accordingly, it is reasonable that by 1996, there could be well over a half-million HIV-infected persons in need of some form of treatment. We need to think now about the potential impact of such a large population of HIV-infected people on our medical system and our society more generally.

NOTES

1. The data in Figures 1 and 2 are estimates made by the Centers for Disease Control (CDC) as of October 1989. (Refer to US Centers for Disease Control, Division of HIV/AIDS. *Report of the HIV/AIDS Projections Workshop, October 31–November 1, 1989.* Atlanta: US Centers for Disease Control, January 1990. These estimates have been corrected for reporting delays.) Additional estimates are provided in an upcoming 1990 article by JE Harris "AIDS Incidence and Reporting Delays" in the *Journal of the American Statistical Association.* (These data have not been corrected for underreporting.)

2. Similar slowdowns in AIDS incidence among homosexual men have been observed in England, Australia, and the Federal Republic of Germany.

3. Gail MH, Rosenberg PS and Goedert JJ. Therapy May Explain Recent Differences in AIDS Incidence. *Journal of Acquired Immune Deficiency Syndromes* 1990; in press.

4. Stoneburner RL, Des Jarlais DC, Benezra D, *et al.* A Larger Spectrum of Severe HIV-1-related Disease in Intravenous Drug Users in New York City. *Science* 242:916-919, 1988.

5. Volberding PA, Lagakos SW, Koch MA, *et al.* Zidovudine in Asymptomatic Human Immunodeficiency Virus Infection. *New England Journal of Medicine* 322:941-949, 1990.

6. Creagh-Kirk T, Doi P, Andrews E, *et al.* Survival Experience Among Patients with AIDS Receiving Zidovudine. *Journal of the American Medical Association* 260:3009-3015, 1988.

7. Volberding, *op. cit.*

8. Gail MH and Brookmeyer R. Methods for Projecting Course of Acquired Immunodeficiency Syndrome Epidemic. *Journal of the National Cancer Institute* 80:900-911, 1988.

9. Harris JE. The Incubation Period for Human Immunodeficiency Virus (HIV-1). In Kulstad R, ed. *AIDS 1988: AAAS Symposia Papers,* pp 67-74, Washington, DC: American Association for the Advancement of Science (1989); and Brookmeyer R and Goedert J. Censoring in an Epidemic, with an Application to Hemophilia-associated AIDS. *Biometrics* 45:325-335, 1989.

10. The details of the statistical method are given in Harris JE, *op. cit.,* note 1.

11. Morgan MM and Curran JWG. Acquired Immunodeficiency Syndrome in the United States: Current and Future Trends. *Public Health Reports* 101:459-465, 1986; US Public Health Service. Report of the Second Public Health Service AIDS Prevention and Control Conference. *Public Health Reports* 103:(Suppl. 1):1-9, 1988; and US Centers for Disease Control, *op. cit.,* note 1.

12. See note 1, *supra.*

13. US Centers for Disease Control. Human Immunodeficiency Virus Infection in the United States: A Review of Current Knowledge. *Morbidity and Mortality Weekly Report* 36(S-6): 1-48, 1987; US Centers for Disease Control. AIDS and Human Immunodeficiency Virus Infection in the United States: 1988 Update. *Morbidity and Mortality Weekly Report* 38(S-4): 1-38, 1989. The decline in HIV incidence is seen in cohorts from San Francisco, Washington, DC, New York, Los Angeles, Baltimore, and Philadelphia.

14. Doll LS, Darrow W, O'Malley P, *et al.* Self-reported Behavioral Change in Homosexual Men in the San Francisco City Clinic Cohort. Abstract F.8.1, p 213, *III International Conference on AIDS.* Washington, DC, 1987; Darrow W. Behavioral Changes in Response to AIDS. *Symposium International de Reflexion sur le SIDA.* Paris, 227-230, 1987; Doll LS and Bye LL. AIDS: Where Reason Prevails. *World Health*

Forum 8:484-488, 1987; McKusick L, Wiley JA, Coates TJ, *et al.* Reported Changes in the Sexual Behavior of Men at Risk for AIDS, San Francisco, 1982-84: The AIDS Behavioral Research Project. *Public Health Reports* 100:622-629, 1985; Winkelstein W, Samuel M, Padian NS, *et al.* The San Francisco Men's Health Study. III. Reduction in Human Immunodeficiency Virus Transmission among Homosexual/Bisexual Men, 1982-86. *American Journal of Public Health* 76:685-689, 1987; San Francisco Department of Public Health. Rectal Gonorrhea in San Francisco, October 1984-September 1986. *Epidemiologic Bulletin No. 2,* San Francisco, December 1986.

15. May RM and Anderson RM. Transmission Dynamics of HIV Infection. *Nature* 326:137-142, 1987.

16. Harris JE. Improved Short-term Survival of AIDS Patients Initially Diagnosed with *Pneumocystis carinii* Pneumonia, 1984 through 1987. *Journal of the American Medical Association* 263:397-401, 1990; Lemp GF, Payne SF, Neal D, *et al.* Survival Trends for Patients with AIDS. *Journal of the American Medical Association* 263:402-406, 1990.

17. Harris, *op. cit.,* note 16.

18. Lemp, *op. cit.,* note 16.

LIVING WITH AIDS

Buddy Clark

I contracted the HIV virus in 1983 and was diagnosed with AIDS in 1984. During the past six years, I've spent much time learning about AIDS, anticipating the disease's progression in my life, and preparing for death. I have made decisions about how my property and possessions should be distributed after my death and, with legal assistance, have executed my will. My funeral arrangements are all in order. Now that I have come to terms with many end-stage issues, I am free to concentrate on living.

I took Amplegin for two years, and I've been on azidothymidine (AZT) for 14 months. Since the beginning of February, I have cut my medication dosage in half. And now I'm beginning to feel like I have a future—it may be short, but I do have one. Recently I bought a new car, and the salesman wanted to sell me a seven-year warranty. I told him I didn't think I needed one. But I'm starting to ask myself the question, what if I do live another five years? I try to focus on staying alive today.

And at LifeLink, that's our message—that AIDS can be a manageable, chronic disease if people take control of their lives, make health preservation decisions, and receive early diagnosis and treatment services. LifeLink, the People With AIDS (PWA) Coalition of Washington, DC, is part of the National Association of PWAs. We seek to empower people with AIDS and HIV infection by encouraging their use of AIDS-related health care and social services. Our case manager helps people that are HIV-infected and their significant others to receive the supportive services they need, including individual and group counseling, legal assistance, housing, drug treatment, food delivery, and information about Social Security and Medicaid benefits. The LifeLink approach to case management is unique in that we help individuals set a series of goals and objectives to meet their anticipated needs while working towards personal change and self-actualization.

At LifeLink, we see education as a vaccine—and we provide comprehensive AIDS education. If people hear and retain the message about safer sex, we're convinced we *can* reduce the number of HIV transmissions. Through our Speakers Bureau, we've reached more than 500,000 people through presentations to churches, schools, businesses, and social organizations, as well as through radio and television appearances. We believe that, in addition to reducing transmission, education will increase everyone's awareness of the disease and reduce fear and discrimination towards people with AIDS.

At LifeLink, we try to support those with HIV infection in many ways. We have a Birthday Club, through which people can ask that donations be made to LifeLink in lieu of birthday gifts. This money is used to help people living with AIDS. Through the Nalley Fund, we also provide direct emergency funding of up to $250 at a given time to help with rent, utilities, food, clothing, transportation, health insurance, prescriptions, or other emergencies. For the approximately 450 babies and toddlers with AIDS living in the Washington, DC, area, we co-sponsor along with the Red Cross a drive for much-needed items—clothes, blankets, diapers, baby food, and toys.

I look forward to the future and my continued work with LifeLink in its mission to "help fight AIDS through information, education, and service."

Buddy Clark serves as the acting president of the Board of Directors of LifeLink, which provides services to people with AIDS (PWA) as the PWA Coalition in Washington, DC, and is an affiliate member of the National Association of People With AIDS.

OVERVIEW OF THE CONTINUUM OF NEEDS AND RESPONSES BY COMMUNITIES

The Robert Wood Johnson Foundation AIDS Prevention and Services Program: A Community Approach

Edward N. Brandt, Jr., MD, PhD, and Deborah Lamm, MPA

☐ Questions and Answers

The Robert Wood Johnson Foundation AIDS Health Services Program

Mervyn F. Silverman, MD, MPH

The Robert Wood Johnson Foundation AIDS Prevention and Services Program: A Community Approach

Edward N. Brandt, Jr., and Deborah Lamm

Introduction

In February 1988, The Robert Wood Johnson Foundation announced a call for proposals for its AIDS Prevention and Services Program. This represented the Foundation's recognition of the need to support education and service initiatives.

Over 1,000 applications were received, with most submitted by community-based organizations. The total requested funds exceeded $500 million. This response is one measure of the enormous need perceived by communities. After careful review, 54 projects were awarded for a total of $16.7 million in December 1988.

From these facts, three observations can be made. First, there is a great need for both prevention and service activities. Second, a large number of organizations are available to perform these activities. Finally, AIDS prevention and service activities are expensive, and, as we shall see, difficult to carry out.

Design of Program

When the AIDS Prevention and Services Program was designed, the goal was to encourage community organizations to study their local needs and to develop approaches to challenge and address those needs. By not dictating program duration, scope, targets, methods, or funding levels, the most creative approaches could be permitted to flourish. What was desired were real solutions to tough problems from people on the front lines. The proposals we received and the proposals we were able to fund covered all the bases.

Descriptions of Projects

In December 1988, The Robert Wood Johnson Foundation approved the 54 grant awards. The funded projects represent a panoply of institutions, services, targets, methods, dollar amounts and commitments of time. In cost, they range in size from $5,000 to $1.8 million. Their duration extends from 12 months to four years. They cover the map from Alaska to Puerto Rico; from Manchester, New Hampshire, to Bartlesville, Oklahoma, and, of course, from San Francisco and Los Angeles through Dallas to New York City, Washington, DC, and Trenton, New Jersey.

Support was provided to hospitals, to national organizations, to fledgling community agencies and to established local AIDS organizations. Project work includes counseling, food distribution, developing

Edward N. Brandt, Jr., MD, PhD, the director of The Robert Wood Johnson Foundation AIDS Prevention and Services Program, is executive dean of the College of Medicine at the University of Oklahoma Health Sciences Center and former assistant secretary for health, U.S. Public Health Service. Deborah Lamm, MPA, is the deputy director of the Foundation's AIDS Prevention and Services Program and formerly served as assistant executive director of the U.S. Conference of Mayors.

drop-in centers for people living with AIDS, referral services, medical care, creating videos and educational programs and so on. Some projects were very risky, and that was known in advance. However, it was also known that AIDS could not and would not wait for proven approaches. This disease demanded that risks be taken.

The projects use multiple service approaches to reach adolescents, mothers and children, Hispanic men, prostitutes, people living with AIDS, IV drug abusers and teen runaways, among others. Working through traditional service settings (such as health clinics), less traditional settings (such as schools), and even less traditional settings (such as theaters, roadside billboards, and outdoor powwows), a wide variety of approaches are being tried, many of them innovative.

Now, one year later, we are trying to put this huge initiative into perspective—for funders, for service providers, and, most importantly, for people living with AIDS and those whose lives are now touched or will soon be touched by this disease. The project sites in operation have been visited, and scores of reports and documents have been reviewed. A few grants have had serious implementation problems. That was anticipated, but virtually all of the projects are performing satisfactorily, and many are demonstrating significant successes.

Nine months into the year, with varying start-up dates, the 54 grantees report a total of more than 900,000 people served: 52,000 by direct services; 847,000 by preventive steps; and 8,000 by a combination approach. Six of these special projects are being presented at this conference. Keep in mind that there are 48 more.

Summaries of Projects

Our sampling of the many different kinds of AIDS prevention and services projects includes:

☐ Over 250,000 cable subscribers in New England are given the opportunity to watch a unique, award-nominated video that deals with AIDS prevention among high school students. The "stars" are students, shown in conversation with a health educator.

☐ Local service groups in Ohio now collaborate in delivering case-managed services to people living with AIDS in a 14-county area around Akron.

☐ Case-managed care is now available to high-risk and HIV-positive clients in a New Jersey methadone maintenance treatment program. A full team of health care professionals follows, treats, and refers almost 300 people monthly.

☐ A community agency in Hartford provides culturally specific educational programs for a Hispanic population, including women, intravenous drug users and gay men.

☐ Volunteer interfaith networks in the South and West are offering counseling, support and assistance to people with AIDS.

☐ The University of California at San Diego is creating a model Management Information System to improve and coordinate care for indigent people living with AIDS who are served by the region's medical community.

☐ The Westchester County (NY) Health Department works with minority youth to create traveling teen theater programs. This grantee was invited to perform at the United Nations on World AIDS Day.

The good news about the AIDS Prevention and Services Program is that we have demonstrated that there is a role in fighting AIDS for every segment of society. In any single community, there is something that can be done by religious organizations, medical groups, public institutions, schools, community agencies, and volunteers. The lessons learned from these projects are transferable, and they can serve as models for other communities.

The picture, however, is not all positive. Here are some of the difficulties that have been encountered:

☐ A few projects were not successful.

☐ High staff turnover rates continue to be common barriers to success in the high-stress field of AIDS.

☐ Everything seems to take a long time, which is frustrating when time is so precious.

☐ AIDS prevention and service activities cost money.

Grant requests for this initiative represent the largest request for funding under any one Robert Wood Johnson Foundation program to date. Yet the funded projects represent barely three percent of national prevention and service funding needs identified by applicants to the Foundation in Spring 1988. This demonstrates that even though increasing amounts of money have been coming from federal, state and local sources, the demand for AIDS services far outpaces available resources now, let alone the future demands of people whose needs are emerging.

Conclusion

Around the country, different stages of the epidemic can be seen. Some communities are already working, some are planning, and some, sadly, are oblivious. Yet, HIV infection and AIDS continue to spread throughout the entire United States.

As concerned professionals, we have a responsibility to all individuals with AIDS, including children, mothers, intravenous drug users, gay men, ethnic minorities, and indeed, all those at risk. We urge you to study carefully the models, experiences, ideas and research findings of special projects like these and then apply them in your community's activities.

The major lesson we have learned from these 54 projects is that there is a role for everyone in the community in dealing with HIV infection and the people living with it. All people have talent that can be used, all people can understand the importance of these efforts, and most people are willing to help.

QUESTIONS AND ANSWERS

Editor's Note: All questions in this section were addressed to and answered by Dr. Edward N. Brandt, Jr.

Q: You served as Assistant Secretary for Health in the Department of Health and Human Services at a controversial time (1981-1984). What is your perception of the approach that administration and the present administration have taken in dealing with AIDS?

A: The present administration is difficult to talk about because I don't know what's happening from the inside. My observation is that on the research side, efforts have been extraordinary. In addition, efforts by the Centers for Disease Control and other prevention efforts are making progress.

This is in great contrast to the atmosphere during the early years of the epidemic, when the issue of whether the disease was God's vengeance created great controversy, and the room would have cleared if someone said they had AIDS. On television, I couldn't use certain phrases to describe how the virus is transmitted, because that might offend the American public, and we had whole meetings about how to refer to sexual intercourse.

Q: If the government had stepped in sooner, what could have been done differently?

A: With the benefit of 20/20 hindsight, I can say it would have been very helpful to have had a blood test in the early days. Getting better public education started earlier would have been very useful, but at the time, we saw that as the role of other public health entities. Until the contamination of the blood supply became evident, it was very difficult to get the message out that AIDS was not strictly a homosexual issue. Then thinking began to evolve, and the public became more willing to listen.

THE ROBERT WOOD JOHNSON FOUNDATION
AIDS HEALTH SERVICES PROGRAM

Mervyn F. Silverman

The AIDS Health Services Program was established by The Robert Wood Johnson Foundation in March 1986 to support projects in the metropolitan areas in the United States with the largest AIDS caseloads. The Foundation funded nine projects in the following 11 cities for four years in two 24-month funding cycles: Atlanta, Georgia; Dallas, Texas; Miami/Fort Lauderdale, Florida; Nassau County/Long Island, New York; Newark and Jersey City, New Jersey; New Orleans, Louisiana; New York City; Palm Beach County, Florida; and Seattle-King County, Washington.

The three major objectives of the AIDS Health Services Program and the nine funded projects have been:

☐ to facilitate the provision of comprehensive and cost-effective health and supportive services to persons with HIV infection

☐ to establish specialized, comprehensive health and supportive services for persons with HIV infection based on the San Francisco model of coordinated, comprehensive health care services. This model relies on the development of case management systems to bring together various service components (practical and psychosocial support and medical care) for persons with HIV infection and AIDS, and

☐ to demonstrate that care can be provided to persons with AIDS more humanely and more cost-effectively by emphasizing alternative, community-based, out-of-hospital care.

Cities with 100 or more cases of AIDS were eligible to be considered for the grants. A major prerequisite was a willingness among medical, social service and community-based organizations to cooperate and collaborate in the development of systems of care. It was hoped that the sites selected would serve as models for similar geographic and demographic areas.

The objectives of the AIDS Health Services Program have been achieved by the grantees with assistance provided by the national program staff at the Institute for Health Policy Studies, University of California at San Francisco, and from the National Advisory Committee, whose members include nationally recognized figures in the field of AIDS care and health policy. During the course of the demonstration program, the Institute staff members have monitored and provided consultation to each of the nine projects on such issues as program implementation, resource development, and modification of goals and objectives to meet the changing nature of the HIV epidemic.

Although the program is based on the San Francisco model of care, each project has been developed to utilize effectively its local public health and community-based organizations to meet the specialized needs of its populations. Below are descriptions of each of the AIDS Health Services Program projects.

Mervyn F. Silverman, MD, MPH, is director of the AIDS Health Services Program and president of the American Foundation for AIDS Research. He serves on the faculty of three universities, including the University of California at San Francisco.

AID Atlanta, Inc.

The AIDS Health Services Program project in Atlanta is administered by AID Atlanta, Inc., a community-based organization that provides emotional support to people with AIDS, as well as practical home support and limited housing on an emergency basis. AID Atlanta's main function within the consortium is in the area of case management provided by the social services department. The case managers coordinate closely with the other subcontractors in the consortium, such as Grady Memorial Hospital and the Visiting Nurses Association of Atlanta. Grady Memorial Hospital provides HIV outpatient services as well as acute care services for persons with HIV infection. The Visiting Nurses Association coordinates home care for people with AIDS and works closely with the emotional and practical support volunteers from AID Atlanta.

In the past year, the Atlanta project has perhaps made the most progress since its inception. It has undergone a complete reorganization and is in the process of reorganizing the case management system. The project has established positive relationships with local community groups, political organizations and agencies.

AIDS Arms Network

The AIDS Health Services Program project in Dallas has assembled a comprehensive consortium that comprises approximately 36 local groups, organizations and institutions. It is one of the largest and most impressive AIDS consortia in the United States, representing most of the major Dallas area religious groups, civic organizations, the University of Texas, Parkland Memorial Hospital, the Department of Public Health, and the local community-based AIDS organizations in the gay community. The project has developed the AIDS Arms Network as the administrative core of the consortium, providing coordination and a well developed, sophisticated, comprehensive, centralized, community-based case management system. The case managers at AIDS Arms Network coordinate with services at Parkland General Hospital, the Visiting Nurses Association, the AIDS Resource Center, and the People With AIDS (PWA) Coalition of Dallas. The PWA Coalition has developed one of the most unique housing programs in the United States.

In this last year of the demonstration program, the Dallas project is in the process of establishing its independence from the Community Council of Greater Dallas. The project remains well organized and managed, and there is evidence of good proactive planning for continuation of the project after the end of Robert Wood Johnson Foundation funding. (See p. 57 for a more complete discussion of the Dallas AIDS Arms Network.)

AIDS Health Services Program for Miami and Fort Lauderdale

The AIDS Health Services Program project in South Florida is one of two double-city projects within this national demonstration program (along with the Newark/Jersey City project). It is administered through the Public Health Trust of Dade County (Miami). The Public Health Trust operates Jackson Memorial Hospital, the largest public health care institution in the southeastern United States. After the New York City project, the South Florida project is the largest and is extremely complex. South Florida has a very diverse ethnic and racial mix in general, as well as within the AIDS population.

The majority of services to persons with AIDS currently are administered from Jackson Memorial

Hospital in Miami. The hospital has a pediatric and adult AIDS outpatient clinic as well as pediatric and adult inpatient units. Community services are coordinated through the local Visiting Nurses Association and Health Crisis Network, a local community-based organization. The Broward County component of the project operates separately and coordinates with the Public Health Trust. Most of the services in Broward County are community-based through Project One in Fort Lauderdale and administered through the local public health unit.

The Miami/Fort Lauderdale project is growing rapidly and reflects the current trends in the epidemic concerning changing issues and populations. The new project director demonstrates the qualities of good planning and leadership for the future.

Nassau County AIDS Care Consortium

The Nassau County AIDS Health Services Program project is administered through the Nassau County Health Department at Nassau County Medical Center. The Medical Center has an outpatient clinic and a modern, spacious inpatient unit. Patient care services tend to be centralized at the Medical Center, with home care contracted out to the Nursing Sisters, a local visiting nurse association. The Long Island Association for AIDS Care (LIAAC) is the community-based organization that provides a wide range of services to all of Long Island, including education, emotional support, case management and support groups.

The Nassau County project has shown evidence of proactive planning for continuation of the project after the end of Robert Wood Johnson Foundation funding. However, they will have to work very hard over the next year to keep the consortium intact. (See p. 109 for a more complete discussion of the Nassau County project.)

AIDS Health Services Program for Newark and Jersey City

The Newark/Jersey City AIDS Health Services Program project is the other double-city project along with one in South Florida. It is administered through the New Jersey State Department of Health. New Jersey has a very unique situation with the HIV epidemic. Although this project serves an urban area and is in close proximity to New York City, the majority of cases are in the heterosexual community and involve IV drug users, minorities, women, and children. AIDS can realistically be approached as a family problem in New Jersey. New Jersey has had success in recruiting rehabilitated drug users to work in the program and has done more to create new approaches to education, prevention and treatment among IV drug users than other projects. Recently, they have been able to add long-term care beds to the project.

The New Jersey project has made great progress in the area of long-term care and remains a model for pediatric AIDS programs for the rest of the country. However, the project is facing major challenges in working with the intravenous drug using population.

New Orleans AIDS Project

The New Orleans AIDS Health Services Program project is unique. Administered through the Associated Catholic Charities of New Orleans, it is a medium-sized project that has grown steadily. Catholic Charities coordinates the project and directs the case management system. New Orleans Charity Hospital has an AIDS outpatient clinic and a busy, dedicated inpatient unit. Both Tulane University and Louisiana State

University Schools of Medicine work with the project, a major advantage. Catholic Charities has been successful in working with community-based organizations, such as Hotel Dieu Community Home Care and Hospice, the Visiting Nurses Association, the New Orleans AIDS project, and the gay community. Education and prevention has been the major focus, as has working with minority communities. The organization has also opened a small residential facility and AIDS hospice called Lazarus House.

In the last year of the demonstration program, the New Orleans project will face enormous internal changes as the Associated Catholic Charities begins to phase out its role and the community takes over the administration of the project. While funding has been a critical issue in the Program overall, the New Orleans project has done a remarkable job with the fewest resources.

New York City AIDS Services Delivery Consortium

The New York City AIDS Health Services Program project is administered through the New York State AIDS Institute. The New York City project is the largest and most complex in the Program. New York City has developed a diverse mix of community services, including: the Gay Men's Health Crisis Center; special services for gay adolescents, IV drug users, minorities, women and children with AIDS; the PWA Coalition; education and prevention services; housing; and hospital care. St. Clare's Hospital in Manhattan has become a model for hospitals changing their focus to deal with HIV. St. Clare's provides all levels of care as well as serving all populations, including prisoners.

The reorganization of the New York City project, focusing on three smaller projects in different communities, is working well as the result of the project's strong leadership.

Comprehensive AIDS Program (West Palm Beach & Belle Glade)

The Palm Beach County AIDS Health Services Program project is the smallest of the projects, but very unusual for other reasons, as well. The project involves two completely different populations. One part of the project is located in West Palm Beach, which is on the Atlantic Coast. The HIV population is predominantly white and gay with a growing number of IV drug users. This is also one of the most affluent communities in the United States. Forty-five miles inland is Belle Glade at the edge of Lake Okeechobee. Belle Glade is a rural migrant agricultural community and is one of the nation's poorest places. It has the highest incidence of HIV infection per capita in the United States, with the majority of cases in minorities, IV drug users, women and children.

Comprehensive AIDS Program (CAP) provides case management services and coordinates the West Palm Beach and Belle Glade components of the project. Palm Beach County does not have a public hospital, but several hospitals in the area participate and coordinate their efforts. The local public health department is a subcontractor and operates AIDS clinics in West Palm Beach and Belle Glade. In addition, the county has opened an AIDS unit in its long-term care facility. In Belle Glade, the entire project is run by people from the area. They provide education, prevention and outreach services as well as home care and transportation services. Belle Glade has been able to develop a small, but very effective program for the local community by working very closely with the county public health department.

During the past year, the West Palm Beach project has stabilized, and has worked well with local community and government groups. The major challenge of the project is determining how the two different communities, the coastal and glades communities, will coordinate services in the future.

Seattle-King County Comprehensive AIDS Services Project

The Seattle-King County AIDS Health Services Program project is administered through the Seattle-King County Department of Public Health. Seattle has been able to plan proactively and add resources and components as necessary. The project has grown rapidly and, more than most projects, has been able to anticipate needs and be prepared to handle them as they arise.

Harborview Medical Center and Swedish Hospital provide outpatient as well as inpatient care. Harborview, the public hospital, has an AIDS clinic, and Swedish Hospital, a private hospital, has a clinic, an inpatient unit and a hospice program. The Northwest AIDS Foundation is the community-based organization that coordinates case management, housing, and emotional support volunteer services, as well as coordinating the supportive services of Shanti Seattle and the Chicken Soup Brigade for practical assistance in the home. Seattle has been able to assemble the most comprehensive array of hospital and community-based services in the Program to date.

The project is stable and well administered. The Seattle project remains smooth-running and has been the most successful in dealing with multiple issues such as funding, case management, and housing. Its major challenge will be developing funding sources to continue its high quality of services. (See p. 120 for a fuller discussion of the housing aspects of the Seattle-King County Project.)

Conclusion

Each of these demonstration projects has had both successes and difficulties. In general, the projects have demonstrated that formerly disparate groups can work together, albeit with some disagreements. Although actual dollar savings cannot be ascertained at this time, we believe that a case-managed continuum of care with emphasis on outpatient services is an effective approach to reducing costs—both human and financial—in dealing with this epidemic and, in fact, with other chronic conditions.

Recurrent themes are seen across all programs, including: insufficient housing, rapidly increasing numbers of clients, need for more present and future funding sources, and political conflicts (between community organizations and among community-based organizations and local and state governments). Although these situations reflect local problems, they are actually national in scope and impact and require increased, ongoing federal support.

SPECIAL BURDENS ON INSTITUTIONS: RESULTS OF NEW STUDIES

AIDS and HIV Treatment in our Cities' Public Hospitals, 1987-1988: Preliminary Analysis

Dennis P. Andrulis, PhD

The HIV-testing Policies of U.S. Hospitals

Charles E. Lewis, MD, ScD
Kathleen Montgomery, PhD
Christopher Corey, MA

☐ Questions and Answers

AIDS AND HIV TREATMENT IN OUR CITIES' PUBLIC HOSPITALS, 1987-1988: PRELIMINARY ANALYSIS

Dennis P. Andrulis

The emergence of AIDS as an epidemic in the 1980s has been paralleled by the emergence of new and formidable treatment burdens placed on the U.S. health care system. As the number of those affected by this disease has risen, the mounting costs in dollars and resources expended in caring for these individuals have become glaringly apparent.

As we enter the 1990s, we begin to see estimates that underscore the tragedy of this condition: AIDS has become the sixth leading cause of death among young adults nationwide, according to the Centers for Disease Control. In New York City, the latest data available show that, in 1988, AIDS was the leading cause of death among women 25 to 29, 30 to 34, and 35 to 39; it was the leading cause of death among New York City children ages 1 to 4 during 1987. By the early 1990s only motor vehicle accidents may cost more in terms of medical care for all age groups. We also begin to see more ominous signs that AIDS is becoming a disease of the medically disenfranchised populations of uninsured, underinsured, and poor children, drug users and their families.

Although steps are being taken to expand the scope of services available to people with AIDS and HIV disease, for the most part the locus of care has remained in the hospital. And while more and more hospitals are treating these patients, the nature of the populations in need makes the nation's safety-net institutions the group most likely to treat disenfranchised individuals infected with this disease.

This paper presents preliminary information, based on our 1988 U.S. Hospital AIDS Survey, on 58 members of the National Association of Public Hospitals, which together represent eight percent of the 730 survey respondents for that year. We describe hospital use, characteristics of the patient population, and financing for these large city institutions during 1988. To gain some perspective on changes in the course of treatment and services provision, we compare these results with findings from our 1987 survey. The paper also reports on the number of people with other HIV problems (but not yet diagnosed as having AIDS) treated in public hospitals for 1988 and relates this population to those diagnosed with AIDS, according to the Centers for Disease Control (CDC) definition. A closing section suggests some implications for these 58 providers.

Study Background

The U.S. Hospital AIDS Survey is an ongoing project, conducted by the National Public Health and Hospital Institute, whose purpose is to monitor treatment, financing, and other factors related to caring for HIV-infected individuals. It was initiated in 1986 with participation from the 465 members of the National Association of Public Hospitals (NAPH) and the Council of Teaching Hospitals (COTH), with initial support from The Robert Wood Johnson Foundation (RWJF). The survey has been conducted for

Dennis P. Andrulis, PhD, is the president of the National Public Health and Hospital Institute and vice president for research and policy of the National Association of Public Hospitals (NAPH) in Washington, DC. He directs the ongoing U.S. Hospital AIDS Survey, initially funded by The Robert Wood Johnson Foundation.

two subsequent years, with support from RWJF, CDC, the Agency for Health Care Policy and Research, and the Bureau of Maternal and Child Health and has grown significantly to represent a 1,200-hospital coalition of several associations (the National Association of Children's Hospitals and Related Institutions, the National Council of Community Hospitals, the Catholic Health Association, NAPH and COTH). The results reported herein are based on responses from the public hospitals who are members of NAPH only.

AIDS Hospital Utilization

The 58 NAPH public hospital members reported treating almost 7,800 AIDS patients during 1988, an average of 134 per institution. Their average length of stay was 17.5 days, their admissions and hospital days per patient per year averaged 1.7 and 29.3., respectively.

Comparison of the preliminary 1988 utilization information with 1987 data indicates a slight decline in length of stay but increases in days and admissions per patient per year (Figure 1). Early indications suggest that much of the increase in these measures is related to changes among public institutions in the Northeast. That is, while public hospitals in other parts of the country are demonstrating, in general, modest declines in patient utilization, northeastern facilities are reporting sizable increases in the average number of days AIDS patients were hospitalized during 1988 and the frequency of admissions. In fact, average length of stay increased as well in this region.

These early findings suggest that the hospitals in the Midwest, South and West continue to make modest progress toward containing the per patient-based utilization rates for AIDS patients. However, public institutions in the Northeast continue to encounter the greatest burden. At least two factors may be placing additional stress on providers in this region: a sicker patient population, and the unavailability of alternative placements for AIDS patients treated in the Northeast's public hospitals.

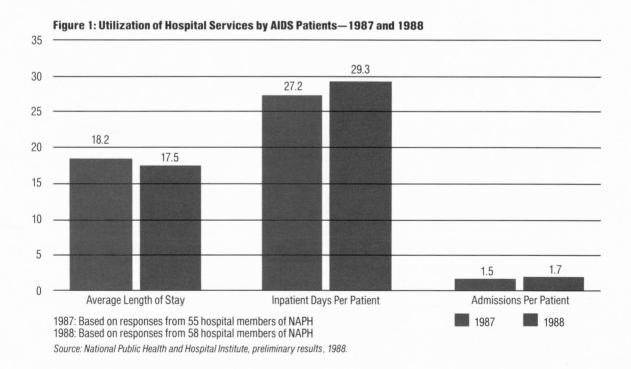

Figure 1: Utilization of Hospital Services by AIDS Patients—1987 and 1988

1987: Based on responses from 55 hospital members of NAPH
1988: Based on responses from 58 hospital members of NAPH

Source: National Public Health and Hospital Institute, preliminary results, 1988.

Comparison of AIDS with Other HIV Patient Utilization

A preliminary comparison of 39 hospitals treating AIDS and other HIV patients indicates that the latter group represents a substantial burden as well (Figure 2). Other HIV patients did not require as many admissions (1.2 versus 1.8 for AIDS patients), and the number of inpatient days per patient per year was almost one-third fewer (22.8 versus 32.9 for AIDS patients). However, the average length of stay for this patient population was only slightly less than for the public hospital AIDS patient (18.3 versus 20.0 for AIDS patients).

These findings suggest that other HIV patients do not need inpatient hospital care at the frequency required by AIDS patients. It does appear, however, that once admitted to the inpatient unit, their illness is sufficiently serious to warrant a hospital length of stay almost equivalent to that of an individual diagnosed with AIDS.

Patient Characteristics

The majority of AIDS patients treated in NAPH member hospitals were, as expected, between the ages of 20 and 49 (90 percent) and male (84 percent). They also continue to be predominantly minority (63 percent), although a slightly higher percent were Caucasian (5 percent) in 1988 compared with 1987.

Risk groups were almost evenly divided between homosexual and other categories. When these 1988 estimates are compared with 1987 responses (Figure 3), it appears that the proportion of AIDS patients classified as homosexual has increased by 10 percent. And, while the total number of heterosexual drug users with AIDS clearly increased, this group as a proportion of the caseload in member institutions decreased by 10 percent.

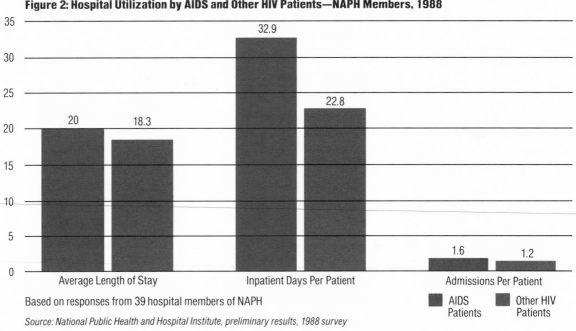

Figure 2: Hospital Utilization by AIDS and Other HIV Patients—NAPH Members, 1988

Based on responses from 39 hospital members of NAPH

Source: National Public Health and Hospital Institute, preliminary results, 1988 survey

While these changes will be examined further in subsequent analyses, one possible explanation could be that many homosexuals who had previously been using private institutions under their insurance policies or with their own funds have now exhausted their benefits or resources. Many also may have become sicker. These situations, especially in combination, may have required these patients to rely on the public hospital system.

Payer Source

A majority of patients treated for AIDS in NAPH institutions during 1988 were Medicaid recipients (60 percent). Combined with the traditional designation for indigent care, i.e., "self pay" or "other" (26 percent), and the very low proportion of privately insured (8 percent), it becomes clear that these institutions treat a very large number of low-income people with AIDS. It is also clear that the proportion of Medicare-paid patients remains low, although Medicare pays for the care of a much higher percent of the general patient population compared to AIDS patients served within these facilities. Thus, it appears that the Medicare "slice of the payer pie" in that general patient population has been replaced by low-income, not privately insured individuals in the AIDS patient population.

The total proportion of primarily low-income AIDS patients (Medicaid, self pay and other) remained very similar between 1987 and 1988 (Figure 4). However, there seems to be a slight shift so that Medicaid is coming to pay for a modestly higher proportion of care for this population. Only marginal changes occurred among other payers, which indicates that Medicare and private insurance continue to play relatively minor roles in NAPH members' AIDS care financing.

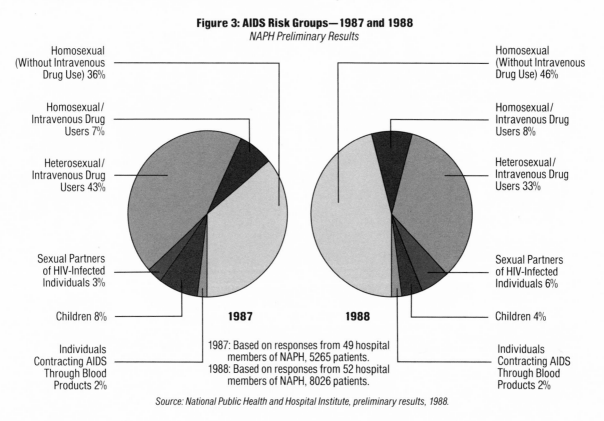

Figure 3: AIDS Risk Groups—1987 and 1988
NAPH Preliminary Results

Homosexual (Without Intravenous Drug Use) 36%

Homosexual/ Intravenous Drug Users 7%

Heterosexual/ Intravenous Drug Users 43%

Sexual Partners of HIV-Infected Individuals 3%

Children 8%

Individuals Contracting AIDS Through Blood Products 2%

1987

1988

1987: Based on responses from 49 hospital members of NAPH, 5265 patients.
1988: Based on responses from 52 hospital members of NAPH, 8026 patients.

Homosexual (Without Intravenous Drug Use) 46%

Homosexual/ Intravenous Drug Users 8%

Heterosexual/ Intravenous Drug Users 33%

Sexual Partners of HIV-Infected Individuals 6%

Children 4%

Individuals Contracting AIDS Through Blood Products 2%

Source: National Public Health and Hospital Institute, preliminary results, 1988.

Summary and Conclusions

Public hospitals represented by the NAPH membership clearly continue to bear an increasing burden of AIDS patients, with the vast majority of these individuals having to rely on public sector support. While many of these facilities across the country seem to be avoiding major increases in utilization, institutions in the Northeast are struggling with a rising use of inpatient beds. Comparison of AIDS with other HIV conditions indicates that, while individual hospitals work to control costly inpatient care, they face a formidable task both in terms of financial requirements and in hospital resources as they struggle to provide services related to the entire spectrum of HIV disease.

To improve this situation would require intensified assistance in shifting the locus of much HIV care away from the inpatient bed to the outpatient and community setting. This shift is desperately needed by many patients as well as providers. Monitoring how well such care is balanced at the community and state levels is also essential if we are to keep public and other institutions from simply being overwhelmed. In some instances, emergency assistance or impact aid may very well be required. Ultimately, however, as we strive to keep pace with the growing number of people diagnosed with HIV-related conditions, we must also consider the changes we must make in our health care system to assure its viability now and in the future.

Figure 4: Inpatient Payer Source—1987 and 1988

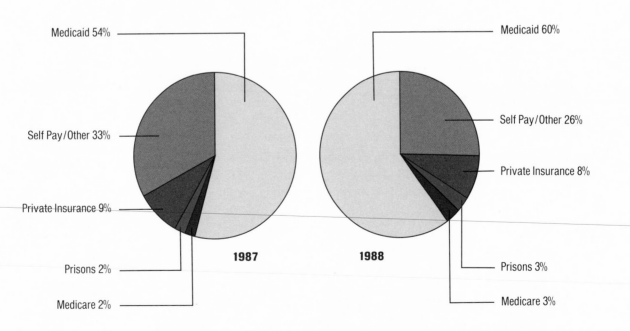

Source: National Public Health and Hospital Institute, preliminary results, 1988.

THE HIV-TESTING POLICIES OF U.S. HOSPITALS

Charles E. Lewis
Kathleen Montgomery
Christopher Corey

Introduction

In July of 1986, the Centers for Disease Control (CDC) held a conference for contractors involved in "community case-finding" studies. At that conference, reports were presented on health workers who had been infected with the human immunodeficiency virus (HIV) due to limited nosocomial exposure. There was an afternoon session marked by vigorous debate about the merits of pre-operative screening of patients admitted to hospitals for the presence of HIV infection. One hospital administrator stated that his board had created a policy requiring all patients to be tested. A surgeon at another institution indicated that his hospital had "solved the problem" of occupational transmission of HIV. All patients were tested: those who tested negative had a green sticker placed on their charts; those who tested positive had a red sticker affixed to their medical records. When asked about patients who refused testing, he responded that they received a red sticker as well. The discussion, or more accurately the arguments, about routine testing of patients admitted to hospitals continued on into the late afternoon.

In August of 1987, the CDC issued recommendations for the prevention of institutional spread of HIV.[1] Included in these recommendations was a brief statement of the conditions under which testing should occur, if in fact the institution chose to pursue this course. The guidelines set forth were quite simple: patients should be informed before testing; patients should be counseled about the meaning of the test before being tested; patients should be informed with regard to the results of their tests; and every attempt should be made to maintain patient confidentiality with regard to the results of the test.

While the debate about routine testing of inpatients continues to swirl around us,[2-4] there have been no data that provide a current picture of the prevalence of policies related to HIV testing in U.S. hospitals. In 1989, we undertook a national survey to obtain such information.

The Pilot Study

The funding agency was justifiably concerned about the degree to which we could persuade hospital administrators and other key spokespersons in their institutions to participate in a telephone interview focused on such a controversial topic. Therefore, we undertook a pilot study in the latter part of 1988 to test a proposed approach to the enrollment of hospitals, as well as to pilot the interview schedules developed for use with chief administrators, directors of nursing, and chiefs of medicine and surgery.

The method consisted of the following steps. First, a phone call was made to the hospital to ensure that the name of the administrator, as listed on the American Hospital Association's (AHA) 1987 data tape, was valid. In fact, a significant percentage of hospitals had changed administrators since the creation of the

One of the authors presented at the workshop. Charles E. Lewis, MD, ScD, is a professor of medicine, public health and nursing at the University of California at Los Angeles.

1987 AHA data tape. Next, an overnight special delivery letter was sent to the administrator by the principal investigator explaining the nature of the study, ensuring confidentiality of responses, and indicating that within 48 hours the administrator would be called by a member of the research staff to answer any questions he or she might have with regard to the survey and to solicit participation. At that time, administrators were to be asked for the names and telephone numbers of the other three respondents within their hospital who could be interviewed.

The initial telephone calls were all made by one of the two primary investigators. This experience gave us some sense of the burden of the questionnaires and surveys that land on the desks of hospital administrators on a daily basis, as well as an awareness of their interest in the topic.

In summary, 80 percent of the hospitals selected at random for the pilot test were enrolled, and interviews were completed with at least three of the four participants at each hospital. This provided sufficient encouragement, and we received approval for the national study.

Sampling for the National Study

A random stratified sample of all U.S. non-federal, short-term general hospitals was selected. The sampling frame included hospital ownership (for-profit, not-for-profit, and public hospitals) and size of the community. We used size of the community as a proxy for the "risk of exposure" of hospitals to AIDS cases. As part of the pilot study, we had obtained a listing of all counties throughout the United States and the number of AIDS cases they had reported to the CDC as of mid-1988. (Since the CDC has only statewide data, data by counties had to be obtained from each of the state reporting offices.) A correlation coefficient of 0.68 was calculated using the size of the county population and number of AIDS cases reported from that county. In addition, not-for-profit hospitals were stratified based on the number of beds—fewer than 200 and over 200.

A total of 716 hospitals were chosen, at random, from the 5,191 hospitals in the universe described. Interviews were completed with three of the four possible spokespersons, including the chief administrator and at least one physician, in 78 percent of these institutions.

Interviewing

The interview with the chief administrator sought data on whether the hospital had admitted a CDC reportable case of AIDS, whether the hospital had a written policy governing such issues as whether patients would be tested for HIV antibodies, or whether the policy specifically forbade testing. In addition, they were asked the year that the hospital testing policy was put into place and, for those institutions without current policies, whether they expected such a policy to be issued within the next 12 months.

Subsequent sections of the interview probed the elements of the policy—whether patients are notified before they are tested, whether they are counseled about the implications of HIV test results before testing, and whether patients are informed of the test results (both positive and negative).

In addition, information was sought as to whether the results of testing are placed upon the patient's chart and who had access to that information in terms of other members of the medical, nursing, housekeeping, and food service staffs. Finally, we asked whether patients who tested positive have their treatment plans reviewed, whether the HIV-positive patients were discharged or transferred elsewhere, and, if so, why.

Information was sought from the administrators as to whether or not staff members had refused to provide care for patients who were HIV positive, and about their awareness of the existence and adequacy of recommendations for testing from a variety of organizations, including the American Medical Association, the American Hospital Association, and the Public Health Service. Information was collected from administrators with regard to time in their current positions as well as their educational background. Data on the characteristics of the hospital were taken from the AHA tape.

In the process of collecting the data, between January and August of 1989, we found very few impediments to completing the interviews. Some hospitals required that we obtain clearance from local hospital counsels; in all cases, such requests were approved.

In 56 percent of the hospitals, interviews were conducted with the chief administrators, and in the others with a deputy administrator selected by the CEO. An analysis of the responses of these two groups of administrators failed to reveal any significant differences.

The interviews were conducted using a computer-assisted interviewing technique by Louis Harris & Associates of New York. Close quality control was maintained, beginning with the training of the interviewers and including periodic monitoring of the quality of the interviews themselves.

In this national study, enrollment was accomplished at the University of California at Los Angeles, and the names and telephone numbers for interviewing were subsequently transferred to Louis Harris. The enrollment process followed in the pilot study was repeated in the national study. It was apparent early on that the principal investigators could not make all of the required telephone calls as follow-up to the overnight letters. Two groups of interviewers were selected to make these initial contacts—retired physicians and professional interviewers who had worked on other hospital-physician surveys. Analysis failed to reveal any difference in the degree of enrollment (or relative success) of each of these two groups, and almost all of the enrollment was accomplished by three physicians and three professional interviewers.

Study Results

An analysis of the data has been completed and has been submitted for publication. We believe we should not present detailed findings at this particular time, since manuscripts are still under review. However, the results generally indicate that the majority of U.S. hospitals, including those in smaller communities, have admitted at least one AIDS patient. A much larger proportion have formal written policies about HIV testing in place, and the growth in the number of those that have policies closely parallels the growth in the number of AIDS cases in the United States. The data, with regard to specific elements of the policies, particularly those aspects or guidelines intended to protect patients' rights, as outlined by the CDC in 1987, are not as prevalent as might be hoped. In fact, there is good reason for prospective hospital patients to ask their physicians whether they will be tested for the presence of HIV antibodies and, if so, what will happen to the test results. Policies in place among hospitals in this national sample do not provide adequate protection of patients' rights.

Note: The research study discussed in this paper was supported through a grant to the University of California at Los Angeles from The Robert Wood Johnson Foundation. Charles E. Lewis, MD, ScD, served as principal investigator, Howard E. Freeman, PhD, served as co-principal investigator, Kathleen Montgomery, PhD, served as project director, and Christopher Corey, MA, served as research associate. Further details regarding the research findings resulting from this study will be published in the future.

NOTES

1. U.S. Centers for Disease Control. Recommendations for Prevention of HIV Transmission in Health Care Settings. *Morbidity and Mortality Weekly Report 36* (25): 1S-18S, August 21, 1987.

2. Hagen MD, Meyer KB, Pauker SG. Routine Preoperative Screening for HIV: Does the Risk to the Surgeon Outweigh the Risk to the Patient? *Journal of the American Medical Association 259*: 1357-1359, March 4, 1988.

3. Rhame FS, Maki DG. The Case for Wider Use of Testing for HIV Infection. *New England Journal of Medicine 320*: 1248-1254, May 11, 1989.

4. Correspondence: Wider Use of Testing for HIV Infection. *New England Journal of Medicine 321*: 1265-1267, November 2, 1989.

QUESTIONS AND ANSWERS

The participants answering questions were, in order of their workshop presentations:

Jeffrey Harris, MD, Associate Professor of Economics, Massachusetts Institute of Technology

Buddy Clark, Acting President, Board of Directors, LifeLink

Mervyn Silverman, MD, Director, AIDS Health Services Program, University of California at San Francisco

Dennis Andrulis, PhD, President, National Public Health and Hospital Institute

Charles Lewis, MD, ScD, Professor of Medicine, Public Health, and Nursing, School of Medicine, University of California at Los Angeles

Howard Freeman, PhD, Professor of Sociology, University of California at Los Angeles

Q: (to Dr. Harris) Please give your interpretation of why there was a slowdown in the AIDS epidemic in 1983-1984 during a time when AIDS wasn't seen as that important by the general public. What has been the role of AZT, of aerosolized pentamidine, and of underreporting in the present slowdown?

A: (by Dr. Harris) Despite the fact that the HIV antibody test didn't appear until 1985, it's likely that among the homosexual community substantial behavior change occurred in 1984. Another explanation may be that the most highly promiscuous people got sick early in the epidemic, and thus there was a slowdown as time went on.

The number receiving AZT in late 1986 and early 1987 was about 8,000. Now AZT is much more widely available. There probably has not been an increase in underreporting. However, reporting is based on inpatient hospital surveillance, and since more patients are being treated on an outpatient basis, cases are being missed.

Q: (to Dr. Silverman) Did you see this rapid behavior change in San Francisco?

A: (by Dr. Silverman) Yes. The fact that there was a huge drop in rectal gonorrhea between 1981 and 1985 reflected a major change in behavior.

Our greatest fears now should be about young people. Somehow, there's a sense that the epidemic is almost over, when in fact the problems will be greatest during the 1990s.

Comment: (by Dallas AIDS Arms Network Director Warren W. Buckingham III) Our volume of AIDS cases has gone from 400 to 1,300, doubling in the last year and a half. We have an increasing number of women among our new cases, so the situation with regard to heterosexual spread is definitely getting more serious from our point of view.

Q: (to Dr. Harris) What are the HIV infection statistics for adolescents?

A: (by Dr. Harris) These data aren't available, but although people with AIDS are out of adolescence, given teens' frequency of sexual activity, the number of partners they may have, and the long dormancy of the HIV virus, we may assume that many cases will be appearing in the future among people infected during adolescence.

TALE OF TWO CITIES: IN-DEPTH ANALYSIS OF RESPONSES TO THE CONTINUUM OF NEEDS

Dallas, Texas:

Developing Coordinated Care for Persons With HIV Illness
Warren W. Buckingham III

The Evolution of an Epidemic: Parkland Memorial Hospital and the New Challenge of AIDS
Ron Anderson, MD

Newark, New Jersey:

Establishing an Integrated Network of AIDS Health Services
Steven R. Young, MSPH, and Adelaide Trautman, MD

☐ Questions and Answers

DEVELOPING COORDINATED CARE FOR PERSONS WITH HIV ILLNESS

Warren W. Buckingham III

Introduction

Less than four years ago, coordinated care for persons with AIDS and other HIV illnesses in Dallas County involved four institutions, four dedicated clergymen, and fewer than 200 persons alive with AIDS. Today, over 40 agencies work through the AIDS Arms Network to provide ongoing services to those with HIV illness, the AIDS Interfaith Network has close to 100 clergy partners as well as 250 volunteers in 17 care teams involved in direct support, and over 2,000 county residents have been diagnosed with AIDS.

While no meaningful "control" has, or could have been, imposed on the growth in the number of cases diagnosed, a comprehensive vision and carefully measured steps have been hallmarks in developing the coordinated care network now in place to meet the needs of those who are ill. The vision is a simple one—*a coordinated approach to service delivery can be overlaid on existing sources of client care without establishing new or redundant service systems.*

The tenets supporting this vision are equally simple.

☐ Voluntary coordination and participation by care-providing agencies is more effective than legislated or litigated "cooperation."

☐ The continuing scarcity of AIDS care resources dictates that participation in a care consortium should not be "bought" as a matter of policy, and non-financial incentives to cooperation must be identified and capitalized upon.

☐ Centralizing and institutionalizing the coordination function—at the individual client and inter-agency levels—is efficient, effective, and yields high-quality results.

☐ While clients served through a coordinated approach (i.e., case management) may consume a wider variety of services than individuals not so assisted, they will use lower levels of high-intensity (and high-cost) tertiary care.

Implementing this vision within the framework of the four tenets above has been the primary responsibility of the AIDS Arms Network over the last 42 months. This paper will review the community-based activities undertaken to establish and sustain a continuum of HIV services in Dallas County and to complement it with simplified access to any and all services through centralized case management.

Needs Identified When AIDS Arms Was Initiated

When the AIDS Arms Network was conceived, services were grouped into three broad categories for planning and organizational purposes: community support, medical care, and in-home and long-term care. The range of services needed to implement a continuum of care and the status of the community's ability to meet those needs was then assessed and is abstracted below.

Warren W. Buckingham III is executive director of AIDS Arms Network, Inc., in Dallas and former associate executive director of the Community Council of Greater Dallas.

Community Support Service Needs

A full array of social support services was deemed essential to the physical and emotional health of persons with HIV illness and their family members, partners, and others. Social support services were also identified to meet needs of professionals and volunteers working with members of the first group and for those who have tested positive for HIV exposure, persons engaging in high-risk behavior, and certain segments of the larger population.

Service needs of the symptomatic population included:

☐ group and individual counseling and pastoral care
☐ direct financial and material assistance
☐ housing
☐ legal assistance, including intervention in discrimination cases
☐ transportation assistance
☐ advocacy for access to all available benefits and entitlement programs
☐ crisis intervention
☐ bereavement counseling for family members and partners, and
☐ assistance in adapting to AIDS-related disabilities (e.g., vision loss or impairment, decreased mobility).

Service needs of the caregiving population included:

☐ stress management assistance
☐ group and individual counseling and pastoral care
☐ risk reduction training
☐ bereavement counseling, and
☐ crisis intervention training.

Service needs of asymptomatic persons, persons-at-risk, and others included:

☐ group and individual educational counseling
☐ group and individual counseling and pastoral care
☐ crisis intervention, and
☐ supportive services in settings other than those principally serving persons associated with risk behaviors.

Medical Service Needs

The following medical services were deemed necessary:

☐ office, clinic, and home-based outpatient care
☐ training and support for physicians, dentists, and allied health personnel so that they dealt appropriately with AIDS/ARC patients and their needs
☐ care with treatment provided by multi-disciplinary teams of health professionals
☐ assistance for physicians, allied health personnel, and others in securing other needed, but non-medical, patient services
☐ access to investigational drugs and treatment protocols, and
☐ local clinical research capability.

In-home and Long-term Care Needs

In addition to assistance with activities of daily living, the following in-home and long-term care needs were identified:

- [ ] a continuum of residential assistance, including cash assistance for rent or mortgage payments, free or low-cost housing for persons with diminished income who are capable of independent living, congregate living for those requiring a more structured setting, and emergency or short-term housing
- [ ] chore and homemaker assistance
- [ ] home nursing services
- [ ] high technology IV and other therapies
- [ ] home health aide services
- [ ] intermediate and skilled nursing home care, and
- [ ] hospice care (in-home, or elsewhere when home death is not appropriate).

Identified Gaps in Services

Needs not being met at the time AIDS Arms was proposed are outlined below. Services not available are differentiated from those where 1986 capacity begged expansion.

Gaps in Social Support Services
Although there were few absolute gaps in social support services for people with HIV disease, it was documented that nearly all in-place programs were at or near service capacity. While volunteers were, and continue to be, the primary providers of support service to patients, the principal organizations recruiting and training volunteers had limited staff capacity to expand and make maximum use of this resource.

Efforts to provide supportive assistance to the caregiving population had been focused primarily on basic education about the syndrome and in-service training for volunteers and some professional caregivers. While informal support groups were being experimented with, plans had not been developed to broaden both the extent and capacity of programs to assist this group.

Although AIDS cases and HIV infection were just beginning to be reported outside the primary at-risk populations in Dallas, a clear need for counseling and other services in settings not primarily identified with the gay community was evident.

Gaps in Medical Services
The following deficiencies in medical services to AIDS/ARC patients were identified:
- [ ] insufficient education and training of physicians, dentists, and allied health personnel regarding care and treatment of AIDS/ARC patients
- [ ] insufficient support for coordination between medical providers and those groups providing the wide range of needed, but non-medical, services to AIDS/ARC patients
- [ ] lack of ongoing clinical research or experimental protocols, and
- [ ] an absence of coordinated assistance for private physicians and others attempting to care for a growing number of indigent patients in both inpatient and outpatient settings.

Gaps in In-home and Long-term Care Services
The principal gaps in in-home services were limited availability of care for persons unable to pay and the unwillingness of any area nursing homes to admit AIDS patients to intermediate or skilled care facility beds. Additionally, in-home hospice care for persons in terminal stages was available only to those who could pay or for the limited number that community agencies were able to support with private donations. No free-standing inpatient hospice care was available.

Strategies Used to Meet Identified Needs

For the needs first identified in 1986, a diverse but complementary set of strategies has been used with good results. These include: aggressively seeking funding to expand or establish needed services; involving "mainstream" service providers in HIV care; and developing greater depth and breadth in local support for an improved response to the HIV epidemic. Details of each strategy are provided below.

Seeking Additional Funding

Since 1986, when the original Robert Wood Johnson Foundation grant was approved, the value of AIDS Arms subcontracts for community services to persons with HIV illness has increased from less than $180,000 to over $1 million. An additional $900,000+ flows to community agencies directly from public sources (the City of Dallas and the State of Texas). No accurate estimate of the increase in private philanthropic support for AIDS work is available, but a conservative approximation puts the 1990 figure at $1 million.

AIDS Arms structured its budget for The Robert Wood Johnson Foundation grant in a way that allowed the agency to wean itself from that source gradually rather than in one lump sum. This has been achieved, as the 1986 operating budget relied on that single source for over 95 percent of its income, but in 1990, the Foundation's grant represents less than 17 percent of the agency's projected income. As the budget has grown, so has the diversity of funding sources. AIDS Arms now has grants or contracts with the city, state, and federal governments and the United Way of Metropolitan Dallas.

The growth in AIDS Arms funds subcontracted for services has been the direct result of successful applications to the Health Resources and Services Administration of the U.S. Public Health Service and the Texas Department of Health. The number of subcontracting agencies has grown from two to 10, and the variety of services supported has similarly expanded. Service priorities are determined and allocation of financial resources is decided through a collaborative process that is facilitated—but not controlled— by AIDS Arms. In the most recent instance, no "set aside" for AIDS Arms case management or administrative expenses was made, and the agency competed on a level field with other providers for a portion of the grant funds to be available from the Texas Department of Health.

As additional dollars have become available from the sources identified above, priority has been given to meeting needs identified in the process of writing the original Robert Wood Johnson Foundation grant proposal. Services now available include: clinical dental care for persons with HIV infection; subsidized housing operated by the Persons with AIDS Coalition of Dallas; an adult day care facility; facility-based day and foster care for children affected by HIV; and significantly increased transportation options. Additionally, the Visiting Nurses Association of Texas, which had some $60,000 available for indigent AIDS patient care in 1985-86, will have close to $1 million available for this purpose in the 1990 fiscal year.

Involving "Mainstream" Agencies in HIV Care Through Case Management

AIDS Arms has deliberately and aggressively pursued participation by the broadest possible array of agencies in community care for those with HIV illness. In just over three years of operation, the number of agencies formally affiliated with the Network has grown from 16 to over 40, and another 30 to 40 agencies are regular sources of assistance with Network clients.

This growth has been possible because no one has been brow-beaten or in any way forced to come to the table. Agencies are invited to enter the coordinated care network at whatever level is feasible within the constraints of corporate mission, budget, and other factors. No agency so invited has declined to participate, and the depth of their involvement has invariably grown over time. The overlaying of case management on this network of care has also played a critical part in the investing of mainstream agencies in AIDS care.

Case management has typically been either medically modeled or practiced within the framework of traditional social work. In the former case, a case manager's primary emphasis is on securing home health care to permit earlier-than-usual discharge of a hospital inpatient. Medical case managers are often registered nurses, are usually employed by hospitals or private insurance carriers, and their activities are in large part driven by cost containment considerations.

The social work case management approach generally deals with community-based clients in specific categories, such as the mentally retarded or mentally ill, or frail and vulnerable elderly people. Master's-level social workers usually fill these positions, and they work for "systems" agencies such as Mental Health/Mental Retardation Authorities which have a legally mandated responsibility to meet the needs of a particular client population.

Because persons with AIDS or other HIV illnesses present such a broad range of social and health care needs and have not (as a class) been legally "assigned" to any systems agency, the Dallas case management program was designed with deliberate departures from traditional models. Therefore, the Dallas model reflects an effort to provide the best of both approaches and fill the gaps in the two. The case management system operated by the AIDS Arms Network has several distinctive features:

☐ Case management is centrally administered, rather than being delivered through positions contracted to other agencies.

☐ A network of formally affiliated provider organizations has been formed to reinforce agencies' commitment to serving persons with HIV illnesses.

☐ Affiliates participate in weekly meetings and/or expedited referral protocols to facilitate provision of service for especially difficult or multi-problem clients.

☐ Typical degree requirements (RNs, MSWs) were set aside to expand the candidate and experience base of potential case managers.

☐ Case managers are called **care coordinators** in an effort to emphasize care for, rather than management of, people in difficult life situations and to minimize confusion based on others' varying definitions of case management.

Case management, or care coordination, is sometimes criticized by those who see it as representing a cost over and above the cost of other services. The Dallas experience to date offers the following responses to that critique.

☐ Centralized case management institutionalizes compassion. Service-giving staff of the AIDS Arms Network are responsible only for seeing that clients' needs are met. They don't say no because "their" counseling slots are full or the food bank is low or the financial relief fund is empty—they find another provider. And they follow up to be sure the client got what was needed.

☐ Centralized case management is cost-effective. AIDS Arms's first three years of operation yielded a unit cost of less than $575 per client. All a care coordinator need do is get a client released from the hospital one day early to "earn" more than it costs to provide case management from the point of intake to death. The savings associated with the Network's increasing ability to prevent some hospitalizations altogether make case management even more valuable to the community.

☐ Centralized case management, which includes weekly meetings of a network of affiliates, provides irreplaceable opportunities for mutual support, with the sharing of both successes and failures among people working day in and day out in the midst of the epidemic. These same meetings also provide a setting for face-to-face contact which builds trust and cooperation among organizations.

☐ Weekly network meetings are Dallas's "AIDS care braintrust," and in that setting creative solutions to what at first appear to be insurmountable problems are quickly developed and remembered when a similar problem arises weeks or months later.

Improving Local Support for Response to the HIV Epidemic

AIDS Arms has followed two routes in improving the local response to the HIV epidemic. First, special efforts have been undertaken to develop a strong, representative, and influential Board of Directors. Second, a great deal of volunteer and staff time and talent were lent to the work of the county-sponsored Dallas AIDS Planning Commission. Additionally, mutually beneficial relationships were cultivated with local media and especially with the editorial staffs of the two Dallas daily newspapers.

Effective community work in Dallas relies heavily on credibility and relationships. A new social or health service enterprise must develop both in short order if it hopes to have staying power. AIDS Arms has achieved this by inviting recognized and dedicated individuals to serve on its Board of Directors and become its representatives to the community. It was initially possible for AIDS Arms to attract people who might not otherwise have agreed to serve on an AIDS Board because it was a project of the Community Council of Greater Dallas, a United Way agency with a solid reputation. Sustaining and expanding this strength on the Board has been a major objective and contribution of AIDS Arms Board leadership.

During 1987, the Dallas County Commissioners' Court convened an AIDS Planning Commission that ultimately involved over 115 citizens in eight working groups. Staff and Board members from AIDS Arms actively endorsed establishment of the Commission and participated heavily in its work. During the planning process, a number of new—and unexpected—"AIDS activists" were identified. Several of those individuals now serve on the AIDS Arms Board of Directors and have played key roles in helping shape the agency's and the community's response to the HIV epidemic. The support lent by AIDS Arms contributed to the final report of the AIDS Planning Commission endorsing case management within a continuum of care and recommending that "AIDS Arms Network should be designated as the agency providing case management in Dallas County." The report also urged "increased funding to support additional staff at the AIDS Arms Network."

Although follow-up action on the total report has been disappointing, AIDS Arms has been able to capitalize on many of the recommendations relating to its operation and role in the community and has acted on them as vigorously as resources have allowed.

Positive change in community attitudes and responses have also been pursued through proactive media relations. Dallas is fortunate in that no local media outlets have sought to sensationalize the HIV epidemic, and AIDS Arms has sought to acknowledge that fact. Additionally, special efforts have been made to inform editorial columnists and editorial boards of both daily papers fully about AIDS in greater Dallas. These efforts have yielded positive results in terms of endorsements of AIDS Arms's positions and, more importantly, a sympathetic response to the plight of persons with AIDS.

Major Accomplishments to Date

In addition to the previously detailed growth in funding, positive media relations, and the strong board which it has developed, AIDS Arms claims the following accomplishments:

☐ securing the *pro bono* assistance of an internationally known management consulting firm in developing concrete plans for long-term success as an independent agency

☐ managing exponential growth in caseload, funding, and staff without losing sight of the underlying principles outlined in the introduction to this document *and* without significant attrition in staff or Board membership, and

☐ being cited with increasing frequency as a model approach to coordinating care for persons with HIV illness through centralized case management.

AIDS Arms was fortunate during 1989 to receive several hundred hours of in-depth consultation from McKinsey & Company in dealing with a lack of common vision among professional and volunteer leadership. The company also provided great help in making and implementing comprehensive plans for successful independence for AIDS Arms as it prepared to leave the "nest" of its Community Council origins. With this assistance, all participants in the Network now are in agreement that the AIDS Arms Network represents this community's decision to face responsibly, effectively, and with compassion the health crisis of HIV illnesses and that it will attempt by coordination of effort and resources to meet the urgent needs of men, women, and children who suffer their ravages.

Emotional exhaustion, or "burnout" among staff and volunteers is frequently cited as a chronic problem for AIDS service organizations. This has not been the case at AIDS Arms, and it is believed that formalizing some common sense approaches to caring for staff has been the major contributor. A professional from outside the agency provides two hours of clinical supervision twice monthly for caregiving staff, with a special emphasis on grief and stress management. Adequate and accessible supervision for service personnel was built into the organizational structure and budgeted. Finally, all staff are regularly involved in strategic planning retreats so that they have a sense of ownership about corporate direction and can focus, for a time at least, on the future rather than the overwhelming present.

AIDS Arms has been cited or presented as a model approach to coordinated care for those with HIV illness in numerous regional and national forums. Further proof of this success is the recent awarding of a $282,000 case management pilot project contract to AIDS Arms by the Texas Department of Human Services, which complimented the agency on having submitted the "perfect application." Every effort is made to share candidly all the lessons learned in the community to date, including its major problems, described below. Given the scarcity of time, funds, and other resources available to those seeking to respond to the HIV crisis, agency management feels obliged to help others avoid its mistakes and not reinvent wheels that roll quite well.

Problems Encountered

In addition to the previously mentioned lack of agreement on the part of volunteer and staff leadership on a vision for the agency, AIDS Arms has encountered several difficulties that may be instructive to other communities. These have included:

☐ investing all expansion funding in service growth for too long a period of time without similar growth in administrative infrastructure

☐ seeking unanimity when consensus would more than suffice, and

☐ failing to adopt formal positions on policy, funding, or service issues with sufficient frequency.

During its first two-and-one-half years of operation, service-providing staff at AIDS Arms grew from three to 11 full-time equivalents, and a volunteer corps of 40 individuals was trained to support additional clients. In the same time period—and only at the tail end of it—administrative staff grew by one position, which represented a 100 percent increase. While detractors are inevitable when "overhead" grows, failure to provide adequately for agency management can and usually does lead to multiple crises. These can include, but are not limited to loss of confidence or interest on the part of the Board; failure to be sufficiently accountable to funders or the general public; revenue shortfalls; and a lack of strategic plans or vision, or worse. AIDS Arms addressed this problem just before it became too late and now has an administrative complement adequate to its responsibilities to clients and the community.

Staff and Board members at AIDS Arms have invested countless hours in seeking to nullify, pacify, or otherwise accommodate a perennial detractor. Upon reflection, the value of a critic or critics can be appreciated, but should not be overreacted to. As stated above, every resource—from time to money to personnel—required to cope with the HIV crisis is in short supply, and it is inadvisable and irresponsible to invest too much of any of them in seeking unanimous approval for an agency's actions when a clear and overwhelming consensus of support exists.

AIDS organizations are regularly called upon to express opinions on funding, public policy, and other issues. If agencies have sufficient credibility, these "opinions" can affect the future in material ways if recast as formal positions with the full weight of corporate policy. Establishing a process whereby the Board is regularly involved in reviewing and adopting official stands on key issues guarantees that volunteer decisionmakers are well informed and fully prepared to advocate the agency's stance. If this is not done, the agency runs the risk of having staff and Board representatives deliver inconsistent messages or even contradicting one another.

Expectations for the Future

AIDS Arms, like every similar agency, has a somewhat unpredictable future. Prospects for continued funding from the federal government are very difficult to gauge at present. The call for early intervention becomes louder each day, but no reliable sources of support for the increased services that call will generate have been identified. As AIDS/HIV move more and more aggressively into populations that have been marginalized by our society, public support for a compassionate response will be more difficult to secure.

Communities like Dallas have developed coordinated responses to AIDS which, while they may vary in configuration and efficacy, have relied in significant measure on the Health Resources and Services Administration (HRSA) of the U.S. Public Health Service for financial support. The Administration's 1990 and 1991 budgets woefully underfund the 25 existing programs and make no provision whatsoever for implementing the HIV service plans being developed—at HRSA's behest—by lower-incidence states and municipalities across the country.

The Centers for Disease Control, through "America Responds to AIDS," is launching a vigorous campaign promoting early intervention for those with asymptomatic HIV infections. AIDS Arms currently declines ongoing service to asymptomatic individuals and has no foreseeable capacity to change that restriction. Similar limitations exist at many other service sites across the country. Beyond community support services, though, where are the plans to provide funding for AZT (Retrovir) for the tens of thousands of uninsured individuals whose life expectancies can be materially extended by its use?

This question leads logically to the remaining challenge the future holds. Increasingly, persons being diagnosed with AIDS or other HIV illnesses come from the neglected underclasses of American society. Who will advocate for the intravenous drug user with HIV? Or the prostitute, or the homeless alcoholic, or the chronically mentally ill persons "deinstitutionalized to the streets" with no ongoing support?

Comprehensive AIDS service agencies like AIDS Arms have the capability to meet the challenges of the second decade of this epidemic, as they've met those of its first decade, but only if they have reliable support for their coordinating and caregiving activities.

The Evolution of an Epidemic: Parkland Memorial Hospital and the New Challenge of AIDS

Ron Anderson

Introduction

When the first case of acquired immune deficiency syndrome (AIDS) was diagnosed in Dallas County in 1981, the disease was a Phase I illness: an acute, untreatable condition that rapidly progressed to death. Since then, effective but expensive advances in therapy are transforming AIDS to a Phase II stage: a more manageable, though still incurable, chronic illness, which, like cancer or end-stage renal disease, requires long-term and expensive treatment.

AIDS patients at Parkland Memorial Hospital and elsewhere are living much longer. Prior to the availability of current treatment, 60 percent of AIDS patients died within one year of diagnosis. Nationwide, that rate has been reduced to 40 percent. At Parkland, it has been reduced to 30 percent.

Because of the aggressive use of such therapies as zidovudine, or AZT, and, particularly, aerosolized pentamidine, pneumonia is no longer the most common cause of death in AIDS patients at Parkland. Only six of the 439 AIDS patients treated in the hospital's AIDS clinic in 1989 died of *Pneumocystis carinii* pneumonia—a relatively rapid killer.

Mycobacterium-avium-intracellular (MAI) infection now is the principal killer of AIDS patients at Parkland. MAI is a tuberculosis-like organism and is the primary cause of the so-called "wasting" syndrome, a relentlessly progressive condition that causes death approximately six months after onset. Even though MAI may be rendered treatable or preventable within two years, equally devastating AIDS conditions remain to be conquered, including cytomegalovirus infection, which causes blindness and dementia, resulting in almost complete dependence on others.

Although medical science is lengthening the lives of AIDS patients, the disease is incapacitating them over longer periods. The trend will require greater dependence on social services and case management more than ever before.

Patient Profile

Each month, approximately 1,300 patients suffering from AIDS or infected with the human immunodeficiency virus (HIV) are treated at Parkland Memorial Hospital's AIDS outpatient clinic. The majority are Anglo homosexual males. Compared to the majority of patients treated in New York-area hospitals, relatively few of Parkland's AIDS patients are intravenous drug abusers. However, just as the number of homosexual AIDS patients began with small numbers in the early 1980s, small, but increasing numbers of women, children and minorities are infected through IV drug abuse. Approximately 150 women have been treated at Parkland so far.

Ron Anderson, MD, is the president and chief executive officer of a public hospital, Parkland Memorial Hospital, in Dallas, Texas, and he is also professor of internal medicine at the University of Texas Southwestern Medical School in Dallas.

Parkland Memorial Hospital is the only public hospital in Dallas County, Texas, a 983 square-mile area with a population of approximately 2 million people. Parkland is the primary teaching hospital of The University of Texas Southwestern Medical School and is the region's primary Level I Trauma Center. Each year, Parkland admits approximately 40,000 patients and delivers about 15,000 babies—making the facility the third-largest birthing hospital in the nation.

The hospital also handles nearly 550,000 patient visits annually in its 144 outpatient clinics and emergency room. In an effort to reduce these numbers, the hospital is establishing a system of Community Oriented Primary Care health centers to bring educational, preventive and public health services into neighborhoods suffering high rates of illness and death. The goal is to reduce the volume of acute and chronic illness from diseases and health problems such as cancer, hypertension, teenage pregnancy, drug abuse and AIDS. These centers are likely to be key primary-care treatment points for many future AIDS patients.

Like most public hospitals throughout the nation, the burden of caring for AIDS patients falls on Parkland, where the majority of all patients, including AIDS patients, are indigent. Approximately 50 percent of all AIDS patients in Dallas County are treated by the hospital, in addition to increasing numbers of AIDS patients from outlying counties that don't have public hospitals.

Case Management Approach

On any single day, approximately 20 AIDS patients are hospitalized at Parkland. Except for hospitalization for acute AIDS-related infections, most patients are seen on an outpatient basis. Medical treatment is augmented by a strong, central case management program. The focus of case management is to develop a continuum of care through wide participation by many health care and community-based agencies. As patients' illnesses progress and they become more dependent, case management assures they receive help for not only medical, but also emotional and financial problems.

Case management eases the transfer from private to public care for patients who have lost their jobs and medical insurance or have exhausted their health insurance benefits. It also increases patients' independence and functional capacity by coordinating the most appropriate care at the most effective and cost-efficient level.

Financing Deficits

One of the greatest handicaps in addressing the AIDS epidemic is the lack of vision of local and state governments. The penuriousness of Texas Medicaid programs is crippling for anyone in need. For example, a family of four must earn less than $3,872 annually to be eligible for Medicaid. The Texas Legislature additionally is unwilling to pay for treatment of diseases it says are caused by personal choices that violate state sodomy laws. As a result, Medicaid reimbursement for treating AIDS patients remains almost nonexistent, even though the costs of care can range from $25,000 to $100,000 over a patient's lifetime. Although local officials are more supportive, financing recommendations by the Dallas County AIDS Planning Commission have remained shelved since its report was published in June 1988.

Parkland, which is operated by the Dallas County Hospital District and receives approximately 55 percent of its operating budget through local property taxes, has been alone among local governmental entities in implementing an active strategic plan to address the epidemic. But funding is limited to available resources. The strategy calls for careful assigning of resources and manpower—a task made more difficult since Parkland already is operating at functional capacity and is a teaching hospital with a closed-faculty program. (Parkland cannot hire clinicians or use private physicians to meet AIDS services demands without the medical school's endorsement and granting of a faculty appointment.)

Organization of Patient Care Services

During the initial stages of the epidemic, a subspecialty clinic—manned principally by infectious disease, immunology and allergy specialists—was established to treat AIDS patients. This clinic was quickly shifted to a primary care model, similar to that found at San Francisco General Hospital. Discharge planning also was implemented to decrease unnecessary hospitalizations. The overall plan included an extensive educational program for hospital employees and the public to reduce exposure to the AIDS virus.

Patient census data was shared with the county health department to develop an AIDS registry so resources could be shifted according to changes in the growth curve of the epidemic. Throughout the treatment program, physicians in the hospital's AIDS outpatient clinic have cooperated with private physicians in treating patients. A natural outcome of this has been increased numbers of private physicians willing to treat AIDS patients. In the beginning of the epidemic, less than a dozen private physicians treated AIDS patients, but great improvement has been made since then; now approximately 40 private physicians are doing so in Dallas County.

The overall strategy coordinated outpatient/inpatient services while linking patients to community services that Parkland does not provide. More than three dozen community-service agencies offer help to AIDS patients through the AIDS Arms Network.

Parkland developed a medical information system of computerized records so physicians could improve collection and monitoring of data to enhance patient services and document research. This has been an important element in registering public health information with the county health department's patient registry. The hospital's internal case-management program complements those of community organizations in linking patients to residential facilities, visiting nurse services, meals on wheels and other needs. The team approach is more humane in that it assures each patient access to a comprehensive level of care that recognizes his or her own value system.

Many of our initial goals have been achieved, including overcoming a backlog of AIDS cases and managing care in a more systematic way. Now, the hospital's Board of Managers has approved a more formal strategic plan and allocated resources for continuation of existing programs while exploring ways to expand and strengthen the continuum of care for AIDS patients in Dallas County.

Outpatient Care and Community Services

The AIDS Outpatient Clinic fills an enormous community need for medical care. Its current caseload of approximately 1,300 patient visits per month requires a disproportionately large share of hospital resources. The cost of treating AIDS patients at Parkland was more than $6 million in 1989—approximately three percent of the hospital's total operating budget.

Most of the clinic's patients are male, but the need for a special maternal-child health clinic became apparent as the number of AIDS and HIV-infected women and infants increased. The hospital responded by establishing a clinic where mother and child can be seen together.

The working relationship with the AIDS Arms Network, the lead case-management organization for community-based agencies, is fine-tuned on a continuing basis. This networking of resources frequently attracts the support of the private sector. The accounting firm, Ernst & Young, recently completed a *pro bono* hospice feasibility study for AIDS patients—Homeward, Inc. Such cooperation also improves the chances that Dallas will compete successfully for more state or federal grants and philanthropic resources.

Other accomplishments include obtaining a $20,000 perinatal grant in partnership with a private non-profit local agency and a private Dallas hospital, Children's Medical Center. The program's goal is to identify HIV-infected mothers and children among the 15,000 babies born annually at Parkland. Without a program assigned to find and help such individuals, they are likely to go without treatment until the disease advances to an acute level.

A $250,000 grant from the Texas Commission on Alcoholism and Drug Abuse is being used to intervene with pregnant women who are abusing drugs. These women also are frequently at high risk of contracting AIDS through drug abuse and transmitting the virus to their unborn babies. Unfortunately, IV drug abusers remain uninformed about the dangers of AIDS or the educational and health programs that could help them, and this program is designed to alter their high-risk behavior.

Clinical and Biomedical Research

Meanwhile, clinical and biomedical research continue to be important elements of the local effort against AIDS. The joint research between Parkland and The University of Texas Southwestern Medical School includes clinical studies on mycobacterium-avium-intracellular (MAI) infection. The federal Food and Drug Administration has approved a study to determine whether the drug rifabutin can prevent MAI infections. Since MAI causes most deaths among the hospital's AIDS patients, clinical research efforts are concentrated on this infection. Additional research proposals include studying a combination of drugs to attack infections such as MAI, *Pneumocystis carinii* pneumonia or cytomegalovirus retinitis. These efforts and others must continue if Parkland is to maintain a grip on the AIDS epidemic in Dallas County.

In forging new programs, it is important to be aware of the many barriers that can block timely response and allocation of resources. Efforts must be made to urge Texas legislators to increase the state's funding of AIDS health care programs. Cooperation and coordination with many community groups must be continued and encouraged, regardless of past problems. For example, criticism directed toward Parkland Hospital by a local gay rights organization escalated into a lawsuit filed against the hospital in 1988. Although Parkland won the lawsuit based on the court's determination that the allegations were without merit, the controversy caused clear divisions in the community. In this stormy political climate, actions were taken which resulted in the loss of funding for AIDS programs.

Beyond hindering day-to-day operations and sapping staff morale, such divisive controversies can deter local philanthropic efforts and weaken legislative resolve to address AIDS health care and prevention needs. Community groups need to set parochial interests aside and work together toward common goals—something easier said than done.

Projections For The Future

Parkland's future course of action against the coming waves of the AIDS epidemic will be critical. Although Parkland is currently seeing a plateau in the volume of new AIDS patients, the numbers are clearly misleading. The true volume of future cases is hidden, because the county health department's AIDS registry lists only the number of AIDS cases and does not include the number of HIV-infected patients. Two private physician group practices are each treating well over 1,000 HIV-infected patients. Patients are remaining healthier longer before their medical conditions mature into full-blown AIDS. Case loads are also growing because patients with AIDS are living longer, more functional lives.

This is a welcome achievement, but it must not lead to complacency. Dallas County is facing inevitable growth in future AIDS patients whose numbers will include not only Anglo gay males but, increasingly, heterosexual men and women of all races. We must try to stay ahead of the epidemic and adjust the delivery of health care and social services to the needs of these many subgroups of AIDS patients.

A sophisticated continuum of care must be in place when the volume of currently asymptomatic HIV-infected individuals enters the health care pipeline. When the impact of that huge patient caseload hits, the effect will be similar to water erupting from a knotted garden hose.

ESTABLISHING AN INTEGRATED NETWORK OF AIDS HEALTH SERVICES

Steven R. Young and Adelaide Trautman

The goal of the New Jersey State Department of Health (NJSDH) in regard to an AIDS/HIV health care delivery system is to "develop an integrated network of AIDS health services that provides for coordinated acute and community-based care for persons with AIDS/HIV infection (PWAs), their families, and significant others." The issues surrounding this goal can be viewed from four broad perspectives:

- [ ] the *cost of care* to New Jersey's system of health care and service delivery
- [ ] the direct impact on professionals and institutions/agencies that have a *role and legal responsibility* to provide care and treatment
- [ ] the broad spectrum of health and social service *needs* of PWAs, and
- [ ] the *nature of the epidemic* in New Jersey and affected population groups.

The delivery of services to persons with AIDS in New Jersey is complicated by four factors: discrimination, poverty, drug abuse, and homelessness. This is evident in the large percentage of minority drug users who are affected by AIDS and to whom project efforts are primarily directed. AIDS has graphically illustrated the fragmented nature of the health care delivery system in our inner cities, particularly Newark, Jersey City and Paterson. Until fairly recently, the Department's program has not had the benefit of strong local leadership, involvement of minority communities in program development, or development of local AIDS service provider networks.

However, by highlighting a chronology of the development of our State AIDS Service Program and its focus on Newark, a sense of our rationale in dealing with a baffling, disturbing and highly political epidemic will emerge:

- [ ] New Jersey was the first and until recently the only state where intravenous drug users (IVDUs) were the predominant risk group; pediatric AIDS was first diagnosed in Newark. Though there is now a separate state-level Division of AIDS Prevention and Control, AIDS activities were once combined with drug abuse activities.
- [ ] The Division of Alcohol and Drug Abuse is part of NJSDH; drug treatment centers were state-run, and though now divested, maintain a strong relationship with the state.
- [ ] In 1984, a National Cancer Institute seroprevalence study conducted in drug treatment centers indicated that in Jersey City 56 percent and in Newark 42 percent of drug users in treatment were HIV-infected. The message was clear: AIDS was a serious problem in this population.
- [ ] Staff moved quickly to integrate infection control practices into the drug treatment centers, and education and treatment policies were developed.
- [ ] As only 10 percent of the addict population was estimated to be in treatment, it was also crucial to begin efforts to reach and educate the 90 percent of addicts not in treatment. In 1985, the ex-addict street educator program was established.
- [ ] AIDS Coordinators were hired and established the first structural basis for a network of care, similar

Steven R. Young, MSPH, is the director of the Care and Treatment Unit organized under the Division of AIDS Prevention and Control of the New Jersey State Department of Health. Adelaide Trautman, MD, serves as medical director of the Newark Department of Health and Human Services.

to those of Gay Men's Health Crisis and Shanti, although on a much more modest level.

☐ A coupon program was established for immediate drug detox. This program was established because those at-risk, particularly black males, were not entering treatment.

☐ Hospital dumping and access problems were dealt with through NJSDH policies and its uncompensated care program.

☐ Getting out of the hospital proved tougher than getting in, and the continuum of care was first addressed in 1986.

☐ State money for direct services was allocated in 1986 for two ambulatory care clinics, two medical day care centers, 35 residential AIDS drug treatment beds, counseling and testing sites, an AIDS home care unit, mobile health vans, and a pediatric residence.

☐ In 1986, the AIDS Community Care Alternatives Program was established through Medicaid. To date, the program has served 1,250 persons.

While these state-funded programs were being successfully implemented, both the growth of the epidemic and periodic failures of the health care delivery system to meet patient needs suggested that the delivery system for PWAs would need continued expansion and, as importantly, coordination at state and local levels. An opportunity for such growth and coordination came via The Robert Wood Johnson Foundation AIDS Health Services Program.

The NJSDH applied to the Foundation for a grant on behalf of a consortium of over 40 health care and welfare providers in Newark and Jersey City. Consultation with these community-based agencies led to two themes in New Jersey's proposal: the need for a broader range of services and the need for a management system to match PWAs to the services they need at the time they need them. The process begun in preparing the grant application was actually the first time a comprehensive AIDS/HIV needs assessment had been completed in these cities.

The NJSDH, acting as lead administrative agency, has directed funds to health care institutions and agencies seeing a large number of clients with HIV infection and has attempted to move both the political and community organization process so that an environment can be established that is more supportive of the necessary range of community-based services. The provision of services based on need is sometimes difficult with a client population that is roughly 80 percent drug-use related. However, the Foundation funding provided the opportunity to begin development of a system of care that focused on local coordination and case management. Conventional reimbursement systems do not pay for such activities.

In Newark and Jersey City, because PWAs first become known to the health care system at hospitals, drug treatment centers, and—to a limited extent—community health centers, the key to providing a multidisciplinary system of care has been a hospital-based case management system and a set of AIDS services revolving around drug abuse treatment.

There has been a major commitment by the NJSDH to fund direct service and education programs in Newark. Specifically, monies have been awarded for:

☐ AIDS coordinators and ex-addict street educators in drug treatment centers
☐ coupon program outreach efforts
☐ counseling and testing sites
☐ residential, respite, and foster care for children
☐ volunteer buddy support
☐ ambulatory care clinics
☐ medical day care

- [ ] dental clinic
- [ ] home health care
- [ ] residential AIDS drug treatment beds
- [ ] minority outreach and education
- [ ] participation in the Community Research Initiative (a community-based clinical trials program)
- [ ] training for health professionals
- [ ] adolescent outreach and support
- [ ] housing programs
- [ ] long-term care, and
- [ ] mobile health vans.

Agencies in our network have received direct funds from The Robert Wood Johnson Foundation (RWJF) and other sources on their own. Currently, RWJF money represents approximately 15 percent of the financial commitment to AIDS service programming in Newark. Although funding sources have diversified, this demonstration project represents the focal point for local coordination and case management.

There has been rapid growth in the availability of services through a fairly sophisticated network, but unfortunately, not enough to keep pace with the epidemic. When our case management program was first initiated, there often were no services to refer to.

Two features of the New Jersey program should make it of particular interest to policymakers. The first is the location of the case management program in acute care hospitals and its linkage with a community-based system operated under the state's Medicaid Waiver Program. Because a central concern of case management programs is to move care away from acute settings, it may reasonably be questioned whether hospital-based programs will be able to reach that goal. A second issue arises out of the characteristics of the population served. Intravenous drug users, because of their distrust of authority, lack of systematic access to health services, and noncompliance with medical and drug treatment protocols, are believed to be a difficult target for case management. Our data and experience tells us case management can work for this population. During the past three years, the 15 case managers in our project have managed care for 2,404 clients with AIDS/HIV infection.

In pursuing a community-based, case-managed system of care, the principal problems have been related to the rapid increase in caseloads, lack of specific types of resources (substance abuse programs, housing, food, mental health services), and a lack of coordinated local-state leadership that includes broad-based community involvement. On a positive note, we have seen the development of a combination of city task forces (which provide an education function and political link), county service provider networks, and private service ventures supported at upper administrative levels of institutions. A challenge continues in the need for coordination of these efforts and for the joint development of long-range city plans and management decisions by these groups.

The difficulties of dealing with intravenous drug users notwithstanding, the evidence suggests that case management does work with this population. Clients are making earlier contact with the health care system than they were prior to the implementation of the demonstration program, and the incidence of unnecessary hospital readmissions appears to have declined. Forthcoming analyses of hospital discharge data from participating hospitals are expected to lend quantitative support to this observation.

The hypothesis has been proposed that case management promotes cost-effective service delivery. It may be that in Newark, our case management approach has directly resulted in the provision of many services not previously provided, and that this has increased total costs. However, the cost-appropriateness of case management cannot be disputed. It should also be noted that case management has been most successful in dealing with the needs of children and their families, most of which include intravenous drug users. The program developed at Children's Hospital in Newark has been adopted as a model for the creation of a network of regional care centers across the state. These centers also will serve the needs of the children's infected mothers.

In summary, the barriers encountered have been many and of both a broad and deep-seated, as well as a specific nature:

☐ homelessness and displacement
☐ a less healthy population
☐ lack of community and political support
☐ lack of private physicians
☐ existence of an AZT black market
☐ high crime—creating a need for escorts for home care providers
☐ lack of volunteer buddies, and
☐ coordination of HIV and substance abuse treatment.

Our strategy for responding to some of these challenges may be out of the mainstream of normal health care delivery, but it has been necessary because of the unusual combination of AIDS and drug abuse. We have:

☐ paid for aides, rather than use volunteers
☐ hired workers indigenous to the affected populations
☐ provided services through existing drug treatment centers
☐ utilized outreach and drop-in centers as a primary method for identifying at-risk groups and for follow-up
☐ provided services through "health care for the homeless" programs
☐ increased reimbursement for services, and
☐ utilized community health centers as provider sites.

Since the first wave of the AIDS epidemic in other places occurred among gay men, there was often an existing nexus of community organizations that could offer volunteer support for those who developed AIDS. There is no parallel group of institutions oriented toward intravenous drug users in the United States outside of the treatment community. Nevertheless, there are always community-based volunteer agencies of some sort that could be drawn into the planning process; in dealing with many health issues, much support typically comes from these community-based volunteer agencies.

Systems strained before AIDS/HIV are near collapse under the weight of the epidemic. Serious health care personnel shortages exist—especially for nurses, home health aides and those with HIV and substance abuse experience—as do barriers in the ability of HIV-infected persons to gain access to primary health care. Demonstrating the well-documented inverse relationship, the lack of outpatient services is going to feed the more costly inpatient system, further burdening individual institutions and the public systems that pay for the majority of such care. Sadly, much of that acute care is preventable. The NJSDH is currently implementing a statewide treatment and assessment program for prophylactic care that we believe will be cost-effective, but will not be cheap. This project builds on the case management, community-based system of care that was developed as part of the Newark demonstration project. It seeks to put in place those services that assure access to the quality early intervention care called for in the federal Public Health Service recommendations.

Finally, we would observe that the patchwork of service and entitlement programs that has developed in Newark and the rest of New Jersey is an outgrowth of the peculiar mix of free enterprise and welfare-based health care that exists in the United States. Through demonstration monies, we have kept cities from collapsing and have developed creative models that work for HIV-infected populations, including drug users. Medium and low-incidence areas need to develop their models and networks of care now before it is too late. And high incidence areas, like Newark—despite their creative solutions—provide evidence that a systems change that includes a commitment to paying for community-based care is essential.

As Dr. Silverman said at the second annual meeting of The Robert Wood Johnson Foundation AIDS Health Services Program, "We are developing programs that deal with people, process, and partnerships in an arena of politics, poverty, and proliferation." The complications that arise in delivering care to the people who need it, when they need it, could be eliminated if our society were willing to make significant changes in the ways in which it funds and manages the delivery of health care. Most of us have experienced the loss of a friend, co-worker, client, lover or family member to this disease; to some of us AIDS is endemic, rather than epidemic. And it is sometimes difficult to be optimistic about anything connected with AIDS/HIV infection. But if it finally moved our society to consider seriously a national health care plan that would support community-based systems of care, it could make a lasting positive contribution to the welfare of all of us.

QUESTIONS AND ANSWERS

The panelists answering questions included, in order of their workshop presentations:

Warren W. Buckingham III, Executive Director, AIDS Arms Network

Ron Anderson, MD, Chief Executive Officer, Parkland Hospital

Steven Young, Director, Care and Treatment Unit, Division of AIDS Prevention and Control, New Jersey State Department of Health

Additional comments are given by Leighton E. Cluff, President, The Robert Wood Johnson Foundation

Q: (to panel) If case management isn't cheaper, then what's the hook for policymakers?

A: (by Anderson) If AIDS patients can be removed from the hospital setting, other indigent patients can be put in those beds. Policymakers should also consider that case managers are more able to provide care consistent with the patient's value system.

Q: (to panel) If officials in Washington, DC, had the power to do something right now, what would you recommend that they do?

A: (by Anderson) Four things: Fund those providers who are carrying a disproportionate amount of the AIDS case load; expand the provider pool; target adolescents within their value system with preventive education (for example, learn how Hispanics view homosexuality and word the preventive message accordingly); and use federal dollars to target AIDS hot spots, such as areas of high drug use and suburban areas like Long Island where sexually active people don't think of themselves as vulnerable to AIDS.

Q: (to panel) Why isn't the Medicaid waiver option for case management being exercised?

A: (by Anderson) The Texas Medicaid system is archaic, and it was very difficult to get the waiver. Since local government orientation varies widely, we need a *national* health policy. The level of Medicaid a state asks for should be available in direct block grants to the cities where they are needed. The waiver should also be set up so that it doesn't pit one need group against another in vying for the funds.

Comment: (by Buckingham) While the case management approach may not save money directly, it can be a proactive, conservative approach. With early intervention, the patient can be helped to plan in advance on how to utilize existing resources. In addition, through early intervention in the disease process, eventual dependence may be delayed considerably. When COBRA coverage is extended, the patient may never need to move to Medicare or Medicaid.

Comment: (by Cluff) These programs have accomplished something we at the Foundation have sought for years—that is, the ability to provide the comprehensive services that former Secretary of Health, Education, and Welfare Elliot Richardson claimed were needed. You have done this by integrating and mobilizing multiple resources that had previously been fragmented. There's a magic to what you've accomplished, and it should be given the broadest possible exposure nationally.

Comment: (by Buckingham) While this model is very apropos for AIDS care, we should keep in mind that for some inner-city populations, there are no resources to coordinate. Most minority groups have little access to long-term care for any purpose, let alone for AIDS.

AIDS PREVENTION FOR HIGH-RISK POPULATIONS

The Chicago Adolescent AIDS Education Program
Douglas N. Bell

The AIDS-HIV Prevention Program for Migrant Workers
Gail Anne Stevens

The AIDS Prevention/Condom Promotion Project: Applying Effective Behavioral Change Techniques for Safer Sex
Deborah A. Cohen, MD

☐ Questions and Answers

THE CHICAGO ADOLESCENT AIDS EDUCATION PROGRAM

Douglas N. Bell

Introduction

Our task at the University of Illinois Adolescent AIDS Education Program has been to design an effective AIDS educational program for Chicago's inner city youth: a program that would be culturally sensitive to black and Hispanic concerns and that would be applicable to the real-life situations these adolescents face on a daily basis.

Due to the high rates of sexual activity and drug use by adolescents and particularly inner-city adolescents, it was clear that this group was primed to carry the next wave of HIV infection. But from the beginning we were faced with a catastrophe within a catastrophe. First, our targeted schools were located in areas where HIV infection was already on the increase. Second, any prospects for effective AIDS education had to be qualified by the fact that 40 to 60 percent of these inner-city high school students would drop out, and, of those who remained through their senior year, up to half were likely to have attained only a fifth grade reading level. Third, this situation itself was embedded in the reality that 35 to 67 percent of the children attending these Chicago public schools live in families whose incomes are below the poverty line. Finally, these areas were imbued in gang violence and drug-dealing. For some students, getting to school was itself an issue of survival.

We knew that because of the difficult life situations of these adolescents, we could not afford the luxury of rhetoric and moral platitudes. We had to go beyond the sloganism of "Just Say No" and beyond a curriculum that conveyed only factual information. Aristotle reflected in the *Nicomachean Ethics* that he considered purely moral and theoretical knowledge to be empty in comparison to the practical understanding embedded in actual situations. He posited that purely theoretical knowledge of the good will not lead to a good life. With very little adjustment, we could apply this perspective to the practice of AIDS education. Thus, in addition to the primary objective of increasing factual knowledge regarding the causes and prevention of AIDS, it was necessary to enhance this education with real-world situations, strategies of action, practical knowledge and behavioral skills.

Strategies and Objectives

We designed our program with just such a strategy in mind. We sought to have the following effects:
- [ ] to increase adolescents' feelings of self-efficacy with respect to their ability to avoid AIDS
- [ ] to help adolescents acquire strategies to finesse and avoid peer pressure and situations that put them at risk for AIDS
- [ ] to develop an awareness of the human costs of AIDS, and compassion for those with it
- [ ] to provide critical support services to persons with AIDS in inner-city neighborhoods, and
- [ ] to establish a school-community network for AIDS prevention and community service.

Douglas N. Bell is principal investigator and program director for the Adolescent AIDS Education Program, conducted by the College of Education, University of Illinois at Chicago.

These objectives were to be achieved by designing the program so that:

☐ the training focused on more than one level (that is, on beliefs and skills, as well as knowledge about AIDS)

☐ the training effectively utilized significant others (especially peers) as the conveyors and reinforcers of knowledge

☐ the training was active rather than passive and included role playing, discussion groups, multi-media presentations, and community involvement

☐ the skills and knowledge provided through the training was applicable to different life situations, and

☐ the training engaged the adolescents in roles and activities that they perceived as significant in their communities, such as peer counseling and community volunteering.

Our major and primary accomplishment from which all other accomplishments stem is that we have a fully functioning program in four inner-city high schools and that the adolescents who have been participating are highly engaged and committed.

The High School-based Groups

Our first accomplishment was getting our program established in the high schools. Four local public high schools participated in the program: Roberto Clemente High School (primarily Puerto Rican), Benito Juarez High School (primarily Mexican), John Marshall High School (primarily black), and George Westinghouse High School (primarily black). In response to the principals' request, we agreed to limit the focus of the program to the freshman class.

We administered a questionnaire to assess knowledge and attitudes of freshmen at each of the participating schools. When the questionnaire was administered we also recruited students to participate in the training program. We mailed parental permission letters (bilingual where appropriate) to the parents of those who volunteered to participate in the program. Overall, we received fewer than 10 rejections from parents.

We had between 200 and 400 volunteers per school. From those, we selected 60 per school to work in groups of 15. The selection of students was based upon their scheduled study periods. The groups were designed to meet once a week for 40 to 90 minutes. During the spring, we rewarded the core of 114 students who had maintained consistent group attendance. Of these, 60 were able to continue through the summer sessions. We currently have 56 fully trained peer counselors, which is slightly more than the 40 (10 per school) we had anticipated.

The Program Design

The ultimate goal of the program was to give adolescents the knowledge and skills to be peer counselors. This was achieved through the design of the program. Because the content of AIDS education and prevention involves issues of sexual behavior and illicit drug-taking, the design of the program had to take into consideration the cultural sensitivities of the target population and the developmental sensitivities of the adolescents. Thus, the structure of the program was designed to be open and interactive enough to allow the participants themselves to contribute to the content, by placing the issues within the context of their social world. The program also was designed to address the issues of adolescents' feelings of self-efficacy and internal attribution (e.g., self-esteem, locus of control), particularly with regard to their ability to avoid situations that placed their health at risk.

The program utilized a small-group format to provide a "safe" environment for discussion and peer support, which in turn provided reinforcement for the strategies learned through the program activities. These activities were designed to engage the adolescents and to develop their behavioral, social, and critical thinking skills. Specific activities included worldview explorations, games, role plays, focused discussion groups, educational film analyses, popular music analyses, and program ownership activities. The content of these activities conveyed information about the behavior and social circumstances that place people at risk.

Program training was designed to be self-affirming and empowering. By creating and acting out social dilemmas in role plays, students have developed their behavioral strategies and social skills. By discussing the issues in focus groups, worldview explorations, and film and music analyses, they have exercised their critical thinking skills and legitimated their opinions. By creating and developing their own videos, public service announcements, and assorted educational materials, they have gained a sense of control and program ownership. By practicing with cucumbers, they have overcome embarrassment and have gained the specific knowledge and skills to describe and/or demonstrate the proper use of condoms. By conducting their own school-wide educational efforts, they have gained recognition from their peers as experts.

Beyond the primary accomplishment of establishing a functioning educational program in the schools, the adolescents themselves have assisted the program by creating and conducting two noteworthy events: a high school "AIDS Awareness Day" and a televised public service announcement. These efforts have had school and community-wide impact.

First, the spring and summer training culminated in the creation of the educational videos. Then, during the fall, the students worked on an educational public service program for Chicago's cable television audience. The program transformed the four individual school videos into one 45-minute program. The creation of the public service program generated more work for the peer counselors, but it also generated a larger than expected audience to benefit from their training. Although we cannot be sure of the exact viewership, Chicago Access is available through cable in 300,000 Chicago-area homes.

Second, the peer counselors at Juarez High School coordinated a highly successful, school-wide "AIDS Awareness Day" to coincide with the World Health Organization's "International AIDS Awareness Day." They posted their own announcements, conducted a condom-related behavior survey of their fellow students, distributed dating tips for teens, distributed bilingual AIDS education pamphlets for teens and parents, conducted videotaped interviews with teens and teachers on their knowledge and attitudes about AIDS, showed the AIDS education video that they had created during the summer, and recruited volunteers to join the program. They reached over 300 adolescents and recruited more than 40 volunteers. Similar schoolwide awareness days are currently being prepared and scheduled at the three other high schools.

Program Evaluation and Material Preparation

By the end of the last quarter, we had completed the session-by-session evaluation of the program's spring and summer educational activities and the facilitator training activities. Based on the evaluations of effectiveness and student response, individual activities are currently being updated, adjusted and assembled. These will form the program activities for the freshman workbooks and peer-educator manuals. Videotapes of sessions that demonstrate a particular game or other activity are also being reviewed for compilation into a video instruction manual. We are preparing a program management guide for running the program when we are no longer supervising it. We will also be working with the volunteer agencies to develop an adolescent volunteer training guide.

Major Obstacles

Throughout this past year there have been some obstacles to overcome: two related to school administration, two related to the students, and one related to the community organizations.

The first administrative issue concerned a major event this past fall. The Chicago Public School system underwent structural changes with the advent of newly elected parent councils. Any event that involved students who did not already have parent permission had to be reconsidered. Thus, the scheduling of our school-wide activities was postponed until we met with the new councils.

The second administrative issue is related to the first and concerned all the school-wide activities. That is, the procedures for gaining approval from teachers, PTA groups, and assistant principals and the procedures for coordinating dates and times with the schools took more time than the actual events. However, these delays were primarily due to caution about issues involving condoms and "street language." If we are successful in integrating this program into the schools' curriculums, this problem should no longer be significant.

The two obstacles associated with the students seem to be more problematic: basic illiteracy and the seeming lack of male interest. First, because our program is not as dependent upon written materials as are most curricula, we did not expect such a high level of discomfort with exercises involving small amounts of writing or reading out loud. Also, knowledge of basic words used in AIDS education could not be assumed. For example, even though some adolescents could point out that "mutual monogamy" was one useful strategy in the prevention of AIDS, when asked, they could not say what "mutual" meant. In response, we have restructured some activities to be less intimidating and added others to help clarify difficult concepts.

Our second student obstacle was not so much attracting male interest in the program as it was maintaining their participation. We have built in monetary rewards ($25 per quarter) and activities that are active and enjoyable. When asked, the males respond that they enjoy coming to sessions, but the majority of male participants (not all of them) have not been as dependable as the female participants. They either are not in school, forget about meetings, get involved in sports, or otherwise do not commit themselves for any length of time. During the summer, most of the male students reported that they could not participate because they had taken summer jobs. This year the program and students themselves are specifically targeting the male population.

The last obstacle to be overcome was in coordinating activities with community-based service organizations. Limited funding has created an atmosphere of competition in which the community-based organizations feel they are at a disadvantage. Our program is attempting to work with some of the agencies that competed for the very funding we received. Also, because each agency has to demonstrate its unique effectiveness, coordinated efforts may be perceived as compromising their ability to garner continuing funds. In addition, even coordinated activities that will increase their number of volunteers involve some amount of manpower. Thus, working with programs such as ours could be perceived as an additional burden on limited resources. Therefore, this year's task has been to coordinate the students and the service organizations so that their efforts are mutually beneficial and optimally time- and cost-efficient.

The Future

After conducting some preliminary one-on-one meetings with individual community-based service organizations during the fall, we met with several of them to "brainstorm" the possible levels of service the adolescents might be able to provide. From this meeting we decided to try a career-day for the students, wherein the service organizations will all meet together to demonstrate their programs and provide a choice of volunteer activities. A monthly rotational system was also suggested.

Our activities planned for the future include: administering the post-test assessment and recruiting new volunteers; recruiting interested teachers and student-nominated high school personnel for training; meeting with school boards, principals, and teachers to discuss our curriculum recommendations; laying the groundwork for future "localized" advisory boards and determining the costs (if any) of program continuation; and setting up a project demonstration meeting for all interested local high schools that might wish to adopt this program.

The issue of future funding for the program remains unresolved. However, we are currently applying for federal funding for a program to train high school personnel in the necessary knowledge and skills to optimally utilize the program materials and to integrate them into their school curricula. We also envision writing grants with the schools or volunteer organizations once we have conducted a financial needs assessment to determine if supplemental funding will be necessary for transportation, male participation, student rewards, video equipment or volunteer organization supervision.

Summary

To sum up our educational success, we can say that the adolescents in our program may at first stumble when attempting to pronounce nonoxynol-9, but they now possess the knowledge of what it does, the behavioral skills of how to put it to use, and the social skills to insist upon using it. We have already seen indications of this result in their discussions and in their videos. From this we have hope. We also feel we have given the adolescents hope. But hope must be given a future. We do not claim to have an answer for all of their problems, but we are well on our way to developing a program that will provide: through their school and community service, new meaning in their lives; through recognition, self-affirmation and empowerment, renewed motivation for their lives; and through increased knowledge and skills, additional means to preserve their lives.

The AIDS-HIV Prevention Program for Migrant Workers

Gail Anne Stevens

Delmarva Rural Ministries (DRM) is a private, non-profit organization founded in 1972 as a service organization to meet the health and social needs of migrants and seasonal farmworkers in Delaware, the eastern shore of Maryland, and Virginia.

The farmworker population is a culturally diverse group composed of myriad ethnic minorities. DRM's 1989 statistics reflect the following ethnic breakdown: 63 percent Hispanic, 16 percent black American, 11 percent Haitian, and 10 percent other (mostly Central Americans and whites).

Farmworkers cannot obtain access to health services through the usual community channels, due to factors such as low levels of literacy, frequent mobility, lack of transportation, language and cultural differences, and dependency on others. Other circumstances, such as the nature of their work and crowded, unsanitary living conditions in rural areas, compound the problems of their lifestyle.

A major component of DRM's activities is to provide health care and health education for farmworkers and their families through bilingual clinicians, health educators and counselors. These services are rendered not only in the clinics, but extended through outreach to labor camps, schools, and churches. AIDS-HIV prevention has been an expanding goal of DRM's program and has progressed with funding from The Robert Wood Johnson Foundation and the states of Delaware and Maryland.

The three goals of the Delmarva Rural Ministries AIDS-HIV Prevention Program and its accomplishments are described below.

(1) *Conduct a needs assessment of farmworkers and area health and social service providers.*

A culturally sensitive knowledge, attitude and behavior survey was conducted in 1989 with 144 farmworkers of the major ethnic groups. While final analysis is yet to be completed, preliminary results show many misperceptions about the transmission of the HIV virus. When farmworkers were asked by what means would they like to receive more information about AIDS-HIV, the majority replied, "from a health care worker."

In terms of local health and social service providers, several workshops were conducted by DRM staff. Information regarding HIV infection and AIDS was provided, as well as information regarding farmworkers in relation to AIDS.

Because farmworkers already face stigmatization and misperceptions from the local community on several cultural levels, DRM felt it important to orient not only providers whose focus is serving farmworkers, but also those agencies that become involved with farmworkers in a peripheral manner, for example, Casa San Francisco, a shelter and community service organization for farmworkers in Sussex County, Delaware, and a migrant Head Start program in Virginia staffed by day care workers. DRM health care staff also participated on a panel for a teleconference on AIDS-HIV infection, broadcast on the eastern shore of Virginia for local health care providers.

(2) *Assess and develop culturally sensitive AIDS education materials for the farmworker population.*

DRM has developed a pamphlet with pictures and a concise message in English, Spanish, and Creole that is sensitive both to the farmworkers and their various ethnic backgrounds. DRM felt it

Gail Anne Stevens is director of health services at Delmarva Rural Ministries, Inc., and has been involved in the work of this agency since 1978.

important to use pictures, as they are a more tangible way to deliver a prevention message and can be used with those farmworkers who cannot read.

With the assistance of "Partners for Appropriate Technology in Health," DRM staff conducted focus group discussions among farmworkers to pre-test posters. Final posters are to be ready in March of 1990 for dissemination this harvest season.

The focus group discussions proved very useful in developing preventive educational materials. Not only will the posters convey the information that the farmworkers felt was important to learn regarding AIDS-HIV, but their involvement also gave the farmworkers a sense of ownership and responsibility for becoming educated about an important health issue.

(3) *Provide AIDS-HIV education to 80 percent of the population or 2,270 farmworkers.*

Information dissemination efforts and health education programs reached 2,909 farmworkers in 1989. The education process took on a three-fold approach. Pamphlets were distributed through outreach to the labor camps. Displays of HIV information as well as condom baskets were set up at each clinic site. Group educational sessions were conducted at the labor camps and in the Migrant Education School Program.

Second, farmworkers who had questions or wanted further information, as well as those identified by the health care staff to be at potential increased risk, were given further individual counseling. If, after individual counseling, a farmworker elected to be tested, he or she was either provided with further counseling and tested at DRM, if a counselor was available (in Delaware and Virginia), or referred to an appropriate HIV testing site. A total of 113 farmworkers received elective counseling and testing at DRM clinics, of whom six were HIV-positive.

Third, in a mass media approach, a farmworker radio program coordinated through DRM aired an AIDS program in Spanish and Creole, reaching not only Virginia, but also the lower shore of Maryland. It is hoped that these efforts will continue during the harvest season of 1990 and be replicated on another radio station in Maryland. There are also plans to encourage more involvement of the farmworkers in the radio program to increase their sense of ownership in developing the types of programming they feel are important.

Another budding effort in effective dissemination of preventive AIDS-HIV information is an exchange program with health care providers from Mexico, to be conducted in partnership with the Sociology Department of Christopher Newport College. A physician from the Public Health System of Mexico visited three of DRM's clinic sites this past summer. DRM's full-time health education coordinator is currently in Mexico to analyze their AIDS health education activities. Through this exchange, it is hoped that more uniformity in content and continuity of preventive messages regarding AIDS will be developed. This is an important initiative, as many farmworkers seek health care in Mexico when they go back to their home base of Texas.

Barriers to Overcome and Future Goals

While DRM is striving hard to meet its goals of offering AIDS-HIV preventive education to farmworkers and has accomplished much in 1989, there are several barriers or problems that have been identified.

One is that, although most of the farmworkers by now have heard the word AIDS or "SIDA" (in Spanish) and can link the word to a severe health problem leading to death, the concept of the HIV virus and its transmission still remains fairly intangible to most. More time is required to be able to do thorough education, and time is a precious commodity when serving a mobile population whose average length of stay on the Delmarva Peninsula is six weeks.

Another problem is that the majority of the population turns over year-to-year. Therefore, next year's farmworkers may include different ethnic groups new to the United States. This forces providers not only to constantly repeat the same information to new groups, but also to adapt materials so that they are sensitive to those particular groups' cultural backgrounds. Some of the more recent ethnic groups come from Third World countries, where they had never experienced organized primary and preventive health care in the western genre. The fluidity of the farmworker population thus creates the need for continual preventive education and the demand for continued and expanding human resources to provide the information.

Although funding through The Robert Wood Johnson Foundation has ended, DRM will continue its commitment to provide preventive AIDS education to farmworkers who come to the Peninsula. Strategies are currently under consideration that will determine percentages of time health staff will spend in AIDS prevention, as well as in continuing to teach other local farmworker service organizations to educate the people they serve. Another strategy is to teach farmworkers to educate other farmworkers.

Finally, while AIDS prevention in many ways has to be treated as a serious priority, much can be said for its becoming a normal part of preventive health care. Providers should routinely educate their patients to prevent contracting the HIV virus, just as they teach patients heart disease risk reduction or car safety with seat belts. All health care providers need to share the responsibility of AIDS preventive education to meet the existing and continuing challenge that faces each and every one of us. DRM will continue to share this responsibility by disseminating information to the farmworkers it serves.

THE AIDS PREVENTION/CONDOM PROMOTION PROJECT: APPLYING EFFECTIVE BEHAVIORAL CHANGE TECHNIQUES FOR SAFER SEX

Deborah A. Cohen

Background

In the era of AIDS, safer sexual behavior is the only viable alternative for people who find abstinence unacceptable. Patients who acquire other sexually transmitted diseases (STDs) are among the highest risk groups for acquiring HIV disease.[1] Several studies have shown that the most important predictor of STD infection is prior STD infection.[2,3,4] Recidivism among patients who receive treatment and counseling in public health sexually transmitted disease clinics in Los Angeles is as high as 75 percent.[5] Clearly, patients with STDs require more effective educational interventions to encourage use of barrier contraceptives and to encourage limiting the number of sexual partners.

The traditional method for promoting safer sex has been to employ an information-only or fear-based approach in which a rationale for safer sex is presented. The dire consequences of the diseases are discussed and the patients' personal risks calculated. The typical messages have been: if you don't use condoms, you'll get a sexually transmitted disease and either become sterile (from gonorrhea), mentally ill (from syphilis), or die (from AIDS). The information/fear approach has been used for the control of sexually transmitted diseases over the past 40 years with little evidence of success.[6] In fact, there is a burgeoning increase in the incidence of most sexually transmitted diseases—including syphilis, venereal warts, chlamydia, penicillin-resistant gonorrhea, cervical cancer, and AIDS.[7] Other studies have documented that knowledge alone does not influence sexual behavior.[8,9] Even when people correctly assess the risks of unprotected sexual activity, many believe they are personally immune from the consequences.[10]

Minorities, particularly blacks and Hispanics, are disproportionately affected by STDs. Fifty-eight percent of children with AIDS are black and 22 percent are Hispanic, representing respectively 15.1 and 9.1 times the incidence of AIDS in white children.[11] Similar proportions are seen among infants with congenital syphilis: 52 percent black, 36 percent Hispanic, and 9 percent white.[12] Among adults with AIDS, 14 percent are Hispanic, and 25 percent are black—double these minorities' respective representation in the U.S. population—these minorities have three times the incidence rate as do whites.[11] Differences in access to health care and exposure to STDs make minorities more vulnerable to STDs.[13] Research specifically directed at these high-risk groups is urgently needed in order to develop effective primary prevention of unprotected sexual behavior.

Strategies to Meet Needs: The Promise of Primary Prevention

There have been substantial successes in interventions for the prevention of smoking and drug abuse. These have been achieved only after careful study and analysis of respective risk factors. When social

Deborah A. Cohen, MD, is an assistant clinical professor in the Department of Family Medicine, AIDS Education Training Center, School of Medicine, University of Southern California.

influences were identified as the major causes of early smoking, interventions teaching social skills to cope with peer pressure and to correct erroneous perceptions of peer smoking prevalence were developed. These have resulted in a decrease in onset of smoking as high as 50 percent in experimental studies.[14]

Similar work is needed to identify risk factors for the development of sexually transmitted diseases and the social and communication skills necessary for the prevention of STDs. Among youth, many of the risk factors for sexually transmitted diseases are similar to those identified for smoking and drug abuse. The pattern of early intercourse leading to lifetime patterns of promiscuity[15] is similar to the pattern observed for smoking—that is, early smokers tend to become lifetime smokers.[16] The transfer of psychosocial research techniques to the field of sexually transmitted disease could prove fruitful in stemming our present day epidemic of syphilis, penicillin-resistant gonorrhea, infertility, cervical cancer, and AIDS.

The Study Design

A study design was developed utilizing three theory-based approaches successfully employed in drug abuse prevention programs. These approaches are being tested among STD clinic patients, singly and in combination, against a control (nonintervention) population. The three basic constructs are:

☐ SKILLS: help patients become familiar with condoms, and demonstrate how to use them.

☐ SOCIAL INFLUENCES: facilitate discussions about how to get sex partners to use condoms, and role-play these negotiations in a group setting. Emphasize the erotic and sensual aspects of condom use.

☐ ENVIRONMENT: make condoms freely available to patients, who can obtain free condoms from designated local businesses by presenting an anonymous ID card.

Rationale for the Interventions

In addition to effective utilization of these constructs in drug prevention research, there have been studies on condom use which also lend support to their applicability in modifying high-risk sexual behavior.

A survey conducted with over 2,000 STD clinic patients identified lack of experience with and knowledge about condoms as a reason for not using them. Many patients stated that lack of availability at the time they were having relations was another factor.[17] One study investigated the feasibility of distributing condoms to an urban male population. When condoms were freely available, more males said they used them the last time they had sex, and fewer males said they had never used them, compared to when condoms were not freely available.[18] These findings support the skills-based and condom availability interventions.

In the condom distribution study, at least 25 percent of the participants stated that the reason they used condoms was because "the other boys do" or because "the girls want me to." This suggests that it may be possible to establish norms that promote condom use among high-risk populations. In one study, couples were instructed about the erotic possibilities of incorporating condom use into sensuous foreplay which resulted in more positive attitudes toward condom use.[19] These two studies support the employment of a social learning intervention.

Accomplishments of the Study

A skills-based approach was piloted in a public health STD clinic. During nine to 12 months, we identified 97 patients who had registered in the clinic the day the skills presentation was given and compared their reinfection rates to those of about 95 patients who visited the clinic on a day the presentation was not given. Study patients were approximately half as likely to return with a new STD infection.

A social influences approach was implemented among patients registered at another STD clinic in which role-playing how to convince a sex partner to use a condom was emphasized. Over 420 patients were identified—half were study patients and half a control group. We found that over the subsequent six to nine months, men who were registered in the clinic the day of the intervention were significantly less likely to return with a newly acquired STD compared to men not exposed to the intervention.

These data are very promising. However, it is too early to tell whether the present larger scale study of more than 1,000 patients will confirm these early findings. Data on potential mediating variables have been collected, which will help us refine and improve the intervention protocol.

Major Hurdles

One of the major problems confronting public health clinics is that the demand for services exceeds the space and the qualified personnel available to handle it. Office space and areas where health educators might speak with patients confidentially are often unavailable. In our experience, waiting room space for group presentations was not always ideal, and patients were continually coming and going during the educational session. In addition, health educators had to be assimilated into the clinic routine.

For the most part, these problems were overcome. While health department personnel tended to be wary of research efforts that might create an additional workload, the regular clinic staff quickly became more comfortable with the health educators' procedures and were highly supportive of our efforts.

Expectations for the Future

The use of behavioral change techniques in the control of STD and HIV transmission is promising. Further research is indicated to improve the current protocols and to focus on the "core" group of persons who repeatedly acquire sexually transmitted diseases. Our approaches are most successful with persons who are just acquiring their first STD. However, the recidivists are also an extremely important group to reach, because they have ingrained habits and are more resistant to change. With repeated exposures, they are the group most likely to acquire and transmit HIV infection.

Government agencies are generally supportive of condom promotion efforts. Although evaluation of educational programs is expected, funding is frequently insufficient to perform the kinds of analyses that are necessary to document efficacy fully—data collection, chart review, and statistical analyses. In general, funding for secondary and tertiary care supersedes funding for research in primary prevention, which deserves a great deal more attention and investment of resources. Evaluation is crucial, because even the most well intentioned programs may have no impact or, worse, exacerbate problems. In the area of drug abuse prevention research, it has been well documented that an information-only approach either has no impact on behavior or results in increased drug experimentation.[20] Since information-only is the approach used in most school AIDS curricula, its impact on sexual behavior among teenagers should be examined carefully.

The principles which have been successfully used in other areas of behavior modification should not only be applied, as we are doing, to high-risk patients, but also to other young people everywhere. Schools need to be able to develop, implement, and evaluate social influences-based curricula on sexuality. Our society must be willing to collect sensitive data on sexual behavior in order to evaluate the true effectiveness of AIDS prevention programs. Without more information about sexuality and the mediators of sexual behavior, we will be permanently handicapped in the battle against AIDS.

NOTES

1. Haverkos, HW and Edelman, R. The Epidemiology of Acquired Immunodeficiency Syndrome among Heterosexuals. *Journal of the American Medical Association 260* (13):1922-1929, October 7, 1988.

2. Tucker, CW. Gonorrhea Recidivism in Richland County, South Carolina. Centers for Disease Control Report #200-76-0672, September 1977.

3. Brooks, GF, Darrow, WW and Day, JA. Repeated Gonorrhea: An Analysis of Importance and Risk Factors. *Journal of Infectious Diseases 137* (2):161-169, February 1978.

4. Richards, EP and Bross, DC. "Legal Aspects of STD Control: Public Duties and Private Rights." In *Sexually Transmitted Diseases,* Second Edition, KK Holmes, PA Mardh, PF Sparling, PJ Wiesner, *et al.,* editors. New York: McGraw-Hill, 1990.

5. Unpublished data, based upon chart review at Central Health Center STD clinic, November, 1987.

6. Turner, CF, Miller, HG and Moses, LE, editors. *AIDS: Sexual Behavior and Intravenous Drug Use.* Chapter 4, "Facilitating Change in Health Behaviors" pp. 259-315, National Academy Press, Washington, DC, 1989.

7. Goldsmith, M.F. Sexually Transmitted Diseases May Reverse the Revolution. *Journal of the American Medical Association 255* (13):1665-1672, 1986.

8. Kegeles, SM, Adler, NE and Irwin, CE. Sexually Active Adolescents and Condoms: Changes Over One Year in Knowledge, Attitudes, and Use. *American Journal of Public Health 78:* 460-461, 1988.

9. McKusick, L, Horstman, W and Coates, TJ. AIDS and Sexual Behavior Reported by Gay Men in San Francisco. *American Journal of Public Health 75:* 493-496, May 1985.

10. Hansen, WB, Hahn, GL and Wolkenstein, BH. Perceived Personal Immunity: Beliefs about Susceptibility to AIDS. (In press, *Journal of Sex Research*).

11. Acquired Immunodeficiency Syndrome among Blacks and Hispanics. *Morbidity and Mortality Weekly Report 35* (42):655-666, October 24, 1986.

12. Congenital Syphilis—United States, 1983-1985. *Morbidity and Mortality Weekly Report 35* (40):625-628, October 10, 1986.

13. Hahn, RA, Magder, LS, Aral, SO, Johnson, RE, *et al.* Race and the Prevalence of Syphilis Seroreactivity in the United States Population: A National Sero-Epidemiologic Study. *American Journal of Public Health 79:* 467-470, April 1989.

14. Botvin, G. Broadening the Focus of Smoking Prevention Strategies. In *Promoting Adolescent Health,* TJ Coates, A Peterson, and C Perry, editors. New York: Academic Press (1982), 137-148.

15. Jessor, R and Jessor, SL. *Problem Behavior and Psychosocial Development: A Longitudinal Study of Youth.* New York: Academic Press, 1977.

16. Smoking and Health: A National Status Report. *Morbidity and Mortality Weekly Report 35* (46): 709-710, 1986.

17. Darrow, WW. "Acceptance of the Condom as a Venereal Disease Prophylactic," In *Sexually Transmitted Diseases.* L Nicholas, editor. Springfield, IL: Charles C. Thomas, Publisher, (1973), 217-225.

18. Arnold, C and Cogswell, B. A Condom Distribution Program for Adolescents: the Findings of a Feasibility Study. *American Journal of Public Health 61* (4):739-750, April 1971.

19. Tanner, WM and Pollack, RH. The Effect of Condom Use and Erotic Instructions on Attitudes Toward Condoms. *Journal of Sex Research 25* (4):537-541, November 1988.

22. Johnson, CA. Prevention and Control of Drug Abuse. In *Public Health and Preventive Medicine.* J Last, editor. Norwalk, CT: Appleton-Century-Crofts, (1986), 1075-1088.

QUESTIONS AND ANSWERS

Questions were answered and comments were made by the following individuals:

Douglas Bell, Principal Investigator and Program Director, Adolescent AIDS Education Program, University of Illinois at Chicago

Leighton E. Cluff, MD, President, and Paul Jellinek, PhD, Senior Program Officer, The Robert Wood Johnson Foundation

Mervyn Silverman, MD, Director of the AIDS Health Services Program, University of California at San Francisco

B.J. Stiles, President, National Leadership Coalition on AIDS

Q: (to panel by Cluff) While the migrant worker program links AIDS with a total primary care effort, the adolescent AIDS education program focuses specifically on AIDS. Is it proper to focus only on AIDS when the population has a multiplicity of problems? There's a policy issue here—is it more appropriate to take a targeted approach or a comprehensive approach?

A: (by Bell) Both prevention through health care delivery and prevention through education are necessary and act to reinforce one another. Although there is some overlap between what each approach accomplishes, they benefit people in different ways. To place these in competition with one another would be counterproductive.

   While the focus of our program is on AIDS education and prevention, the strategy of assessing and incorporating the social world of the adolescent brings into focus other health risks such as drug and alcohol abuse, teenage pregnancy, and sexually transmitted diseases. Adolescent involvement in creating videos, acting in role plays and in other activities makes health-related issues salient to their experience. Discussions revolving around AIDS prevention help clarify misconceptions adolescents have about their own physiology and the maintenance of their general health.

   I would suggest that policymakers consider the benefits of a well designed educational program targeted on AIDS that makes salient the comprehensive health issues linked to AIDS. We should keep in mind that for these targeted populations, AIDS competes with seemingly more immediate survival issues. Yet, if approached properly, AIDS provides the individual with the sense of urgency necessary to counteract apathy and indifference towards health issues generally and to take health maintenance seriously.

Comment: (not identified) There is commonality with both approaches. The risk with a more comprehensive approach is that the AIDS prevention message will be diluted. With the targeted approach, AIDS prevention education may be used as a point of entry to talk about other important health issues.

Q: (to Bell) What have been the outcomes of your AIDS education efforts with teens? Do you know whether there is behavior change?

A: (by Bell) Our program outcomes concern the impact and effectiveness of various educational activities and media on adolescents' knowledge, attitudes, and interests. State law prohibits our ability to ask minors direct questions about behavior. However, we have been able to ask questions about attitudes toward behavior. Results from these measures indicate behavioral change. In addition, small group discussions have revealed that trained adolescents express attitudes of health advocacy and that they have adopted health maintenance behavior. They have incorporated what they have learned and applied it to their lives.

Examples have been buying condoms for friends and partners who are too embarrassed, integrating AIDS information and behavioral strategies into conversations with friends who confide their sexual activities, and taking the initiative to educate and distribute literature to family and friends as well as neighbors who "shoot drugs" after observing their behavior and lack of knowledge.

Q: (to Bell) With a dropout rate of probably over 50 percent, how do you reach those kids who aren't in school?

A: (by Bell) There are currently three methods of reaching the adolescent dropout population. First, reach them before they drop out. Second, reach them through their social networks with their in-school friends. Or, reach them through community agencies. Since half of high school dropouts occur between the freshman and sophomore years, our program is designed to target the freshman class so that the majority of adolescents can be reached while they are still in school. Also, on an inter-agency level, our program is a member of a coalition of community youth service agencies who educate teens about AIDS. We share information and strategies with one another. These community agencies work out of drop-in centers and conduct AIDS education with both in-school adolescents and dropouts.

Comment: (by Stiles) In the Workforce 2000 agenda, employers are becoming actively interested in how issues like AIDS and illiteracy are affecting present employees as well as the adolescent worker of the future. So AIDS is helping us break new ground and take action—for example, in examining how services are organized and prevention approaches are implemented. However, because the political challenges are enormous, change will probably be incremental.

Comment: (by Jellinek) AIDS is helping us to break new ground and take more radical action than we did in the past—in the ways services are being organized, the ways agencies are networking, and the innovative approaches that are being taken.

Comment: (by Silverman) Both around the country and internationally, I've become more and more aware of how cognizant we must be of the other concerns of the people we deal with. For example, if you are trying to talk with runaway teens about AIDS, you must be aware that uppermost on their minds may be the question of where they're going to sleep that night.

COMMUNITY-BASED AIDS SUPPORT SERVICES

Project Open Hand: Home-delivered Meals for People With AIDS in San Francisco
Ruth Brinker

Teleconference Education and Support Groups for People With AIDS in Rural Oklahoma
Marylee Behrens

Assisting People With AIDS Through Volunteers of Legal Service, Inc.
William J. Dean

☐ Questions and Answers

PROJECT OPEN HAND: HOME-DELIVERED MEALS FOR PEOPLE WITH AIDS IN SAN FRANCISCO

Ruth Brinker

I welcome this opportunity to speak about Project Open Hand and the importance of providing nutrition to people with AIDS. In the words of Dr. Donald Kotler of Columbia University College of Physicians and Surgeons, "nutrition has been the stepchild of AIDS treatment far too long."

For the major part of my adult life, I've felt deeply that if someone with a problem crossed my path, I was morally obligated to help them in whatever way I could. In 1985, I watched a friend die of AIDS. At that time, I knew nothing about AIDS except what I had read in the papers, which wasn't much—just statistics. I was shaken to see how quickly my friend became too ill to take care of himself. (Remember, this was before AZT or any other life-prolonging drugs.) Certainly, he could not shop for or prepare his own meals. While a group of us took care of him until the end, I began worrying about all the other people with AIDS throughout the city who probably did not have my friend's support. Because of them, I felt compelled to begin Project Open Hand.

The Birth of Project Open Hand

In the fall of 1985, working out of the 100-year-old kitchen of Trinity Church, I began preparing meals. I began serving seven people two meals a day, a hot entree and a bag lunch. I wanted the meals to reflect the love I had for my friend, so from the beginning, I aimed to provide only the best possible foods. We use nothing but fresh vegetables; processed foods never darken our door. Because the disease leaves many impoverished, we made the service available free of charge—the Zen Center had given me $2,000, and I felt rich.

I learned later that ours was the first program of this type in the country. Since then, we've helped a number of other programs get started—some becoming virtual clones of Open Hand. Because I had been with the local meals-on-wheels program for about 12 years, I knew how to structure such a service. I am, of course, eager to have meals delivered to people with AIDS wherever the disease exists.

People with AIDS and Malnutrition

In the beginning, I would frequently find people with AIDS on the floor when I finally got to their apartments. They would get out of bed, crawl to the buzzer, pull themselves up to buzz me in and then not have the strength to get back into bed. People would tell me that they would sometimes get out of bed intending to get to the kitchen to find something to eat. However, by the time they got to the kitchen, they were so weak they could only turn around and fall back into bed without having eaten. Stories like this—and there were many of them—convinced me that across the country many people with AIDS were dying, not of AIDS, but of malnutrition.

Ruth Brinker is executive director of San Francisco's Project Open Hand, which she founded in 1985. She had earlier directed both meals-on-wheels and meals for the homeless programs.

Getting sufficient money to keep the program going has always been a major problem, but at the beginning we were constantly on the brink of financial disaster. However, on March 17, 1987, when we were serving 128 people daily and had only enough money to last until the end of the month, the San Francisco *Chronicle* ran a small story with an accompanying photo. Suddenly, I was buried under an avalanche of mail—each envelope containing a check. That was the beginning of our explosive growth and also the beginning of our very good relationship with the media. The media attention has brought us funding. Although, unfortunately, we could use still more. It has also brought us volunteers. We are a primarily volunteer organization. And it has resulted in a rapidly expanding client list.

A New Kitchen and More Clients

In March 1987, we served 128 people. By the fall, we were serving 278, and Dr. C. Everett Koop was warning that the number of AIDS patients would quadruple by 1991. Clearly, our 100-year-old kitchen was not going to be adequate, so we purchased a building. With the help of a grant from Chevron Corporation, a generous bequest, and a saintly contracting firm, we installed a 3,800-square-foot kitchen in a building that had housed a Japanese import/export business.

While work proceeded on the building, the number of clients continued to increase, and we were spilling out of the church kitchen. Volunteers were peeling potatoes and carrots in the hall and up the stairs. My outer office became the sandwich assembly area, the ladies vesting room became the computer room, and the choir room became our bookkeeping department. Before we moved into our new building, we were serving 500 clients 1,000 meals a day.

We made our move on February 14, 1989, without missing a single day's service. In fact, from the day I started the program until now, we have not missed a single day. Even on the day of the earthquake, which occurred halfway through the delivery pick-up period, all of the meals went out. A 7.1 earthquake was not going to keep our volunteers from fulfilling their obligations or our clients from receiving their meals. From the day the program started, no one with AIDS or ARC who has appealed to us has been refused service, and no one has been put on a waiting list. If we are called before 10 a.m., the meals are delivered that afternoon; otherwise, the first delivery is made the following day.

Expansion of Services

I feel an obligation to continually strive to improve our service. To that end, we remember everyone's birthday with a cake; we deliver pet food so that animal lovers will be able to hang onto that kind of unconditional love; we provide a party in a box on New Year's Eve and a bag of gifts on Christmas. Children receive Valentine candy and balloons, and on Easter they receive baskets and balloons.

Again, aiming to improve service, we launched a research program to determine the cause of food aversions in the terminally ill, funded by The Robert Wood Johnson Foundation. Dr. Angela Little, professor emeritus at the University of California at Berkeley, conducts this research. She is also developing a Project Open Hand food supplement so we can provide additional nutrition to people who have trouble with regular food.

From the beginning we offered vegetarian meals for those who preferred them. We substituted fish or poultry for those who did not eat red meat; we served soft or liquid foods for anyone who needed this kind of meal. Through an outreach worker, we have made contact with the minority communities, and our three ethnic chefs can provide Asian, Latino, and Black American foods.

Innovative Approaches to Service and Fundraising

We have nutrition software. We enter each menu into the computer, to be analyzed nutritionally so we can see where the meal is lacking and make an adjustment. This way we can make certain that we are providing all the trace elements and other nutrients people with AIDS need.

While we are one of the newer AIDS projects in town, we are now the third largest. In 1986, our budget for the entire year was $69,000. Our budget for 1990 is $3,000,000. While I have had no experience or training in running a multi-million dollar corporation, I do have a wise board. Early on they saw the need for an experienced chief operating officer and provided one. They also found a chief development officer and support staff.

What I do provide is an instinctive feel for what seriously ill people need to make them feel cared for. I really do care about them, so I function as the heart of the program. I am also a principal fundraiser and creator of new funding sources. Because the AIDS funding dollar is shrinking, and because we don't like competing with our friends for money, we are trying to find ways to become self-sufficient.

The Open Hand cookbook is a case in point. Fortunately, it is selling well throughout the country and has been on our local bestseller list for 14 weeks. We are planning another cookbook to be released in the fall of 1991. We also have various businesses in the planning stages.

Future Plans

Where does Project Open Hand go from here? Since the first of January the program has grown 15 percent. I see the number of people served doubling by the end of the year. I see Open Hand expanding its services to other areas. We have already begun service in the East Bay—Berkeley and Oakland, and we are moving forward to bring the program to Marin and Sonoma counties.

In June, when the International AIDS Conference will be held in San Francisco, we are planning a reception for all agencies providing meals or who have an interest in providing meals for people with AIDS. We will give them a tour of our dream kitchen and present them with a copy of our replication manual, which will soon be available to interested groups. This manual is a step-by-step guide on how to begin and run a meal service operation like Project Open Hand. Combined with an institutional cookbook planned for release early in 1991, we hope these tools will help revolutionize institutional cooking everywhere.

Because we constantly need to solicit contributions of fresh, quality foods, the truck we were recently given will be making regular trips to friendly grocers in the delta region of the bay to pick up large quantities of freshly picked vegetables.

I recently suggested to the national director of the 4-H Club, who is also a deputy director of the U.S. Food and Drug Administration, that since 4-H members were already raising champion-caliber livestock to be shown at county fairs, it shouldn't be much trouble for them to raise an additional ordinary stock animal for meat to be contributed to Open Hand or to other programs serving the destitute and hungry. In this way, members of 4-H could make an enormous impact on hunger in the United States. With the enthusiastic support of the director of the California State 4-H, such a program is getting off the ground rapidly in northern California with many young people eager to fight hunger in this way. Project Open Hand has assumed a life of its own and directs our progress into areas completely new to us. Funding is still precarious, but our recent earthquake brought us to the attention of corporations that had never supported us before, and we hope they will continue to do so.

TELECONFERENCE EDUCATION AND SUPPORT GROUPS FOR PEOPLE WITH AIDS IN RURAL OKLAHOMA

Marylee Behrens

Introduction

For the past year, EduMed Incorporated of Bartlesville, Oklahoma, has been offering a service which has been very successful in helping people with AIDS (PWAs) cope with the challenges posed to them by being HIV-positive and isolated in rural Oklahoma. That service provides telephone support groups and educational programs to PWAs in rural Oklahoma and includes one-third of all Oklahoma PWAs. This paper will cover five aspects of EduMed's project: the needs at the outset, the strategy for meeting those needs, the accomplishments, the major hurdles, and expectations for the project's future.

The Needs of PWAs in Rural Areas

In reviewing what has been learned in the past year of the project and in surveying other Oklahoma service providers and PWAs, it appears that the medical, legal, financial, and psychosocial needs of PWAs in rural Oklahoma are probably similar to what service providers are familiar with in New York or San Francisco, with one important difference.

The difference is the severe limitations on availability of services to meet those needs for PWAs in the rural areas of the state. As with PWAs in other parts of the country, persons with AIDS and HIV infection in rural Oklahoma need access to information about medical services, legal matters, programs offered by the Department of Human Services, and general health information, as well as the very important psychosocial support. Although Oklahoma's two metropolitan areas of Tulsa and Oklahoma counties have services for persons with AIDS, there were no such services for the widely dispersed PWAs in rural areas. Most PWAs in rural Oklahoma have to travel for several hours to Tulsa or Oklahoma City to reach a physician who is knowledgeable about AIDS and willing to treat them. Most find that the caseworkers in their local Department of Human Services office do not know what special assistance is available to PWAs. And most PWAs in rural Oklahoma do not even know one other person with AIDS who is within a hundred mile radius with whom they can share their concerns.

EduMed tried to address the educational and psychosocial difficulties HIV-infected persons face when they live in rural Oklahoma. Of course, traveling to Tulsa or Oklahoma City for AIDS information and a psychosocial support group may have been an option for some rural PWAs, but the long distances and expense made regular travel prohibitive for most of them.

Psychosocial support was felt to be a particularly compelling need for PWAs in rural areas because of the stigma attached to the diagnosis of AIDS and HIV infection. The great majority of AIDS cases (66 percent) in Oklahoma are in homosexual and bisexual men. Since Oklahoma is a strong Bible-Belt state, the public has great disapproval and distaste for this lifestyle. This disapproval, which turns into fear and

Marylee Behrens is the project director of the AIDS Service Project for EduMed, Inc., in Bartlesville, Oklahoma. As a certified AIDS educator and HIV-test counselor, she counsels clients at an anonymous HIV-testing clinic in Tulsa.

rejection, is focused on persons with AIDS, which makes them feel like pariahs. Issues about whom to tell about their diagnosis and when and how to tell them are complex. This decision process is very difficult for most and can be facilitated with psychosocial support. For many PWAs, becoming ill with AIDS forces them—sometimes for the first time in their lives—to contemplate coming out of the closet and admitting to family, friends, and community that they are gay. This decision process is also very difficult for most and can be facilitated with psychosocial support. As their illness progresses, PWAs also need psychosocial support to deal with issues of living with AIDS and with death and dying.

In addition to the need for psychosocial support, many PWAs need access to information about medical, legal, and financial services available to them. Education about health information on such topics as safer sex, nutrition, and stress management is also needed.

To meet these educational and psychosocial needs of rural PWAs, EduMed staff proposed teleconference support and education groups: free, anonymous telephone education and psychosocial support groups in a conference-call format.

Originally, EduMed proposed to serve two groups of nine PWAs, each led by an experienced counselor. These groups were to "meet" every week. Three weeks out of the month, the PWAs would interact with each other, getting to know each other and providing support. During the fourth week, the groups would be addressed by an expert in some relevant area—such as medical, legal, or financial services—to provide education and information.

Successes of the Teleconference Support Groups

In the past year, these goals have been accomplished and exceeded. Although EduMed originally proposed to serve two support groups with nine PWA members each, the service was so much in demand that other groups also were established. In addition to groups for PWAs and HIV-infected individuals, there are now groups for spouses and partners of PWAs and for mothers of HIV-infected persons, as well as a bereavement group for those who have lost a loved one to AIDS. In all, there are five groups with a total of 40 members.

The support groups are anonymous for members. Each group has a facilitator—a psychologist or social worker—or in the case of the bereavement group, a hospital chaplain. The PWA group members come from three main risk groups: homosexual men, bisexual men, and hemophiliacs.

The conference-call format allows up to nine PWAs and one facilitator to be on the line together and carry on a group discussion. The advantage of the support group on the telephone is that PWAs can meet with each other without ever leaving their own home, office, or hospital telephone. A criticism that is sometimes raised by counselors not involved in the project is that the telephone format does not allow for some support group-type activities, such as hugging. While it is true that one cannot receive a hug or be together in person over the phone, the group members do receive tremendous emotional support and understanding.

According to members' reports, the groups have been very helpful. The members report that they had felt very alone and had not had anyone to talk to about the problems related to their diagnosis before joining the groups. Most now report feeling that they have people who understand and accept them and will listen to their concerns.

Challenges of the Project

A major hurdle in the success of this project was locating PWAs in rural Oklahoma. Except for the gay organizations with members in Tulsa and Oklahoma City, there were no established routes to reach rural PWAs to let them know that our service was available. To overcome this difficulty, in the early months of the project, the project coordinator traveled all over Oklahoma to many small towns and rural sites. She spoke with physicians, counselors, directors of county health departments, and citizens' groups. In addition to these networking activities, the coordinator issued press releases to rural newspapers announcing the project and put advertisements in the state's one gay newspaper. The project was listed with numerous social service agencies for referrals and in the State Department of Health's publication, *Oklahoma AIDS Update*.

At first it seemed that the information was not reaching PWAs; then a slow trickle of calls started coming in. About this time, the project coordinator started visiting HIV-test clinics and telling the clients there that the service was available. This "personal touch" seemed to be just the boost that the project needed, and many group members were enrolled. In addition, rural patients of the Oklahoma Hemophilia Center who were HIV-positive were contacted and invited to join a support group.

Moving Ahead

In the future, EduMed expects the demand for this service to continue and probably even to grow as the word reaches more PWAs through the grapevine.

Funding has been secured to continue operations through September 1990. Other sources of funding are currently being sought to continue this project past September. EduMed's ability to meet the current demand for services and the possible expansion of services is dependent upon securing funding to cover the many hours of long distance phone calls involved and the remuneration for the facilitators' many hours of counseling. EduMed wants to continue to provide these support group services that have become so important to the PWAs of rural Oklahoma. As one group member said, "I don't know how I ever made it without my phone friends." At EduMed, we hope that he will never be without his phone friends again.

Assisting People With AIDS Through Volunteers of Legal Service, Inc.

William J. Dean

Need at Outset of Project

Volunteers of Legal Service (VOLS) was formed five years ago with a pledge by law firms and law departments of corporations to provide increased *pro bono* legal services to New York City's poor. We have sought in our work to identify some of the critical social problems facing poor people in New York City and to undertake the more difficult task of identifying areas where volunteer attorneys can work to ameliorate these problems. It would be hard to identify a more needy population than persons with AIDS.

Strategy to Meet Needs

First, to serve AIDS inpatients at hospitals, we decided to match law firms with hospitals—in other words, to request that law firms commit themselves to providing volunteer attorneys on a regular basis at a particular hospital. There are advantages to this approach: the law firm comes to feel a proprietary interest in the project and develops close working relations with the medical staff and social workers; and the volunteer lawyers feel they are part of a team rather than working in isolation in their firm. The same rationale applies to providing legal services to ambulatory persons with AIDS.

Second, we decided to limit legal assistance to certain areas: custody and guardianship issues (advising parents with AIDS as to the best provision that can be made for the future care of their children), wills, living wills, and powers-of-attorney.

For clients with children, their most valuable "possessions," by far, are their children. Clients seeking assistance on guardianship issues are typically women who are single parents. Often the client will want her mother, or a sister, aunt or friend to care for her children after her death. Wills are prepared so that clients can choose which friends and family members inherit their very modest belongings. Living wills give specific instructions to hospital staff on limiting heroic measures in certain circumstances. Powers-of-attorney enable a friend or family member to cash benefit checks and pay rent and other bills on behalf of the person with AIDS.

When a legal problem falls outside of these areas—for example, a housing or immigration matter—VOLS tries to secure assistance through its many contacts in New York City with legal services organizations.

As each new hospital site is brought into the project, VOLS provides assistance in designing intake forms and referral procedures and in organizing orientation sessions for the volunteer lawyers. The sessions cover such topics as the nature of the disease, the special needs of the patient population to be served, and the legal services provided by the program, explained in a way that a lay person can understand. Special attention is paid to sensitizing lawyers to the physical and emotional needs of AIDS patients, many of whom are young and very frightened, to ensure as productive an attorney-client relationship as possible.

William J. Dean has been executive director of Volunteers of Legal Service, Inc., in New York City since 1987. Previously he had a private law practice in New York.

Accomplishments

Law firms recruited by VOLS now provide legal services to persons with AIDS at six hospitals:

Hospital	Law Firms
St. Clare's Hospital and Health Center (Summer 1988)	Dewey, Ballantine, Bushby, Palmer & Wood; Wien, Malkin & Bettex; and a pool of attorneys from other firms
Beth Israel Medical Center (Spring 1989)	Paul, Weiss, Rifkind, Wharton & Garrison
St. Luke's/Roosevelt Hospital Center (Summer 1989)	White & Case
New York Hospital-Cornell Medical Center (Summer 1989)	Sullivan & Cromwell
Columbia Presbyterian Medical Center (Fall 1989)	DeForest & Duer
Cabrini Medical Center (Winter 1990)	Simpson Thacher & Bartlett

Social workers at the hospitals identify persons with AIDS who wish to consult a lawyer. The lead social worker then contacts the lead attorney at the law firm. A lawyer promptly goes to the hospital to see his or her client. (At New York Hospital, outpatients are served at a weekly legal clinic. Social workers inform the outpatients about the program.)

Serving Ambulatory People With AIDS

VOLS also has organized two legal clinics to serve ambulatory persons with AIDS. These are outpatients from various hospitals in the city. This is being done in cooperation with the Division of AIDS Services of the New York City Human Resources Administration (HRA). HRA is the main local government social service agency in New York City. The Division of AIDS Services is responsible for providing Medicaid-eligible persons with AIDS living in the community with various services.

Last spring, working with the Division, VOLS established a legal clinic at the Nevins Center in downtown Brooklyn. Over 30 percent of current Division clients in New York City come from Brooklyn. The law firm of Milbank, Tweed, Hadley & McCloy was matched with the Division's Nevins Center by VOLS. Lawyers from this firm visit the center each week and offer free legal services to clients who have requested assistance. These clients have been identified by their caseworkers.

VOLS started a second legal clinic serving ambulatory persons with AIDS last month at the Division's office in Queens County. The law firm of Weil, Gotshal & Manges is providing legal services at this clinic.

In 1989, a total of 159 clients were served: 113 men and 46 women. Forty-five were white, non-Hispanic; 60 Hispanic; 39 black; 2 Asian; and 13 unrecorded. As an indication of the growth of the program, in the first quarter of 1989, eight clients were served; in the fourth quarter, 59 clients were served. All clients served by the program are poor; all are on Medicaid. About 90 lawyers are now participating in the project.

Major Hurdles

The lawyers have been wonderful—prompt, sensitive, professional, caring. It is exciting to see three professions working together in harmony: medical, legal and social work.

The biggest problem has been the disarray which exists in a number of hospitals in New York City as a result of overcrowding caused by increased poverty, drug use, and AIDS in the city, by labor shortages, and by financial difficulties. The health care system is terribly overstrained. There is considerable turnover among medical and social work staff. Each time this happens, the new hospital team has to be informed about the project.

Social workers carry unmanageable caseloads. Thus, not all patients who may wish to meet with a lawyer hear about this project. Since the hours of the work day are finite, sometimes our project gets lost in the rush of hospital personnel trying to do too many things.

In short, once a match is arranged by VOLS between a law firm and hospital, we cannot walk away from the scene. At some, if not all, of the hospitals, we must—and do—continue to prod the hospital staff to give this program priority.

Expectations for the Future

In New York City, over 23,000 AIDS cases have been identified during the past eight years. Some experts predict that there may be as many as 25,000 new cases over the next two years. An estimated 200,000 New Yorkers carry the AIDS virus. Unfortunately, because of these numbers, the need for expansion of this program is unlimited.

We have begun discussions with officials at Bellevue Hospital. Our plans are to provide this service to the 100 AIDS outpatients served by the Bellevue Methadone Maintenance Treatment Program. This would be our first venture with a hospital run by the New York City Health and Hospitals Corporation. (The hospitals where we now work are all voluntary hospitals.) We plan to expand the program to other hospitals and, perhaps, to other borough offices of the Division of AIDS Services.

As AIDS in New York City involves more and more people living in the poorest communities and increasingly becomes a family disease, we expect to be serving many more women clients with children. At one hospital where we already work, 35 percent of AIDS patients are young women with children.

Conclusion

Through this project, VOLS provides the moral and professional imperative—and the practical means— by which the resources of highly skilled volunteer lawyers are put to use for the benefit of people in great need. Obviously, lawyers cannot affect the course of the disease, but we can afford people with AIDS some peace of mind through counsel on basic legal concerns.

QUESTIONS AND ANSWERS

This was a general question-and-answer period that allowed comments and questions to any of the speakers thus far. The names and titles of those who answered a question are listed here.

Douglas Bell, Principal Investigator and Program Director, Adolescent AIDS Education Program, University of Illinois at Chicago

Deborah Cohen, MD, Assistant Clinical Professor, Department of Family Medicine, AIDS Education and Training Center, University of Southern California

Charles Lewis, MD, ScD, Professor of Medicine, Public Health, and Nursing, School of Medicine, University of California at Los Angeles

Ron Anderson, MD, Chief Executive Officer, Parkland Hospital, Dallas, Texas

Warren W. Buckingham III, Project Director, AIDS Arms Network, Dallas, Texas

Mervyn Silverman, MD, Director, AIDS Health Services Program, University of California at San Francisco

Ruth Brinker, Executive Director, Project Open Hand, San Francisco

Q: (to Bell) It must be difficult to deal with teens. Do you find that the good kid is seen as a wimp and that boys are less likely to come to AIDS education programs? How do you drag them in?

A: (by Bell) Working with teenagers is not a problem and is actually enjoyable once you have gained their trust. The crucial stage is getting the adolescents to volunteer to become a part of the program. We have designed our program to appeal to the majority of the adolescents, not just the "good" kids. Other kids need AIDS education, too, and do not necessarily lack the skills that would make them good peer leaders. We have attempted to attract a variety of adolescents (both male and female) and have combined several strategies to do so. We offer school credit or a small amount of money as a reward. We conduct the sessions during the students' free period, while they are already in school. We use trained peer counselors to recruit. We appeal to their desire to get involved in something different, such as video production. We appeal to their desire to help their community. And, we appeal to their desire to become leaders.

By and large, males have been harder to get invested in the project. Their flexible in-school time tends to already be occupied with either sports or part-time work. Also, they tend to be more resistant or indifferent to AIDS as an issue. However, once they attend the sessions, they become involved in the activities and become committed to the idea of becoming peer counselors. The few males that initially became a part of the program have recruited their male friends. Also, the school-wide AIDS Awareness activities have provided the male peer counselors opportunities to become role models for the other males, demonstrating that knowledge about AIDS is both "safe" and status-enhancing. These are among the key benefits of using a peer-to-peer approach.

Comment: (by Cohen) There's a whole literature on the reduction of drug and tobacco use by teaching students to resist peer pressure and by changing normative expectations. We need to apply these psychosocial techniques to AIDS prevention.

Comment: (by Lewis) When teens become active in their own education they are readily involved. In one similar experiment, teens living in juvenile halls were given video cameras to go out and shoot their experience of the world, and they came back with remarkable footage. Their videos were edited into novellas and used for discussions that were effective because the kids had *lived* the story.

Q: (to all) One of the chief retardants to progress in AIDS education and services has been the conflict among the various groups working with AIDS. How can conflict management be done in this area?

A: (by Anderson) First, those involved have to come to the conclusion that they really have the same end in mind—for example, to establish a better system of care. Then, when conflicts arise, the focus can be on mutually desired outcomes. However, it's a mistake to think that consensus is always required, because there are sometimes people who don't *want* to solve the conflict.

Q: (to all) We are developing many laudable AIDS programs directed to various population groups, and the same is true with drug programs. But are we beginning to create separate health care systems for specific problems, and if so, do we want to continue in this direction, or do we want to merge these programs with the overall health care system?

A: (by Buckingham) Of the 44 Dallas agencies working within the AIDS Arms Network, only four are specifically targeted to AIDS, so I'm not sure this is a valid concern.

Q: (to all) Maybe we're asking if there shouldn't be a spillover effect to other populations—for example, comprehensive health care for the disabled.

A: (by Anderson) I'm for universal health care, but you still have to focus on especially vulnerable populations.

Comment: (by Silverman) AIDS can be mainstreamed, but it shouldn't be normalized, because unlike heart disease or cancer, AIDS is a communicable disease. The public shouldn't jump to the conclusion that because AIDS is becoming more a disease of minorities—blacks and Hispanics—things will get better for the general population. We must put resources into primary prevention as well as services.

Comment: (by Anderson) Right now, AIDS is easy to overlook because four percent of hospitals are handling 55 percent of the AIDS caseload. But the ripple effect will be drastic as the situation worsens for these hospitals. For example, a rural Texas hospital will be unable to send an AIDS patient to Parkland, because our caseload is already overwhelming. If there were a more equitable distribution of AIDS patients among hospitals, then the issue would become that of financing indigent care.

Right now, the healthy and wealthy are overinsured, and the system rewards consumption. We have to ask why the system is set up so that the poor person is valued less than the worker or the wealthy.

Comment: (by Brinker) It seems that we should be able to release federal government disaster funds for AIDS, since it is in fact a natural disaster.

HOUSING AND LONG-TERM CARE FOR PEOPLE WITH AIDS

AIDS: The Suburban Perspective
Gail Barouh, MA

Providing Care in a County Nursing Home AIDS Unit
Shauna Dunn, RN, MS

A Comprehensive Approach to AIDS Housing in a Second-Wave City:
The Seattle-King County Model
Patricia L. McInturff, MPA

☐ Questions and Answers

AIDS: The Suburban Perspective

Gail Barouh

LIAAC's First Year: Our Initial Challenges and Needs

I'd like to start with an observation I made during this past holiday season. At the end of the year, Long Island Association for AIDS Care, Inc., (LIAAC) throws a holiday party for our clients. I remember that, at the first party, in 1987, there were mostly gay People With AIDS (PWAs). At the next year's party, there were more partners and spouses. This year, whole families came, and there were lots of children.

Long Island is experiencing the evolution of AIDS. This experience explodes the myths so many people still hold onto about this disease. At LIAAC, we suspected this would be the case. It's only taken four years to prove our predictions true. Before LIAAC incorporated, in the early to mid-1980s, it was accepted that New York State was the epicenter of this disease, with over one-third of the nation's AIDS cases.[1,2] So it was clear Long Island would be hard-hit by this epidemic.

Long Island is, and always has been, the suburban area with the nation's highest incidence of AIDS. The Centers for Disease Control rank Long Island, which is LIAAC's territory—that is, Nassau and Suffolk counties—number 18 among the 25 cities with the highest incidence of AIDS.[3] This means that, as a suburb, we are counting more AIDS cases than such cities as Detroit and Baltimore.

Let's take a closer look at the Long Island community. Nassau and Suffolk counties cover 1,200 square miles and have a population of 2.6 million. These 2.6 million people are popularly thought of as white, middle- and upper-class nuclear families who commute to good jobs, who go to the beach in the summer, and who park at least two cars in their garages. They'd better have two cars, because Long Island has almost no public transportation.

That simple fact can lead us to look below the rosy surface of suburban life. Transportation, housing, health care, even hunger are problems for a growing number of Long Islanders who don't have the income it takes to keep up. Alcohol and drug abuse are also taking their toll across all social lines. Long Island has many minority populations, including blacks, Hispanics, and gays who are living without much of the recognition and social support found in cities of comparable size. However, AIDS is forcing our social service agencies and local governments to recognize these people because they are the Long Islanders who are shouldering the burden of this disease.

AIDS is a horrible way to get attention, but it's turning the focus on long-overlooked members of the Long Island community, for example:

☐ Blacks represent seven percent of the Long Island population,[4] but constitute 27 percent of our people with AIDS.[5]

☐ Hispanics are four percent of our population,[6] but seven percent of our AIDS cases.[7]

☐ Gay men are estimated to be approximately 10 percent of the area population,[8] and they account for 35 percent of people with AIDS.[9]

Gail Barouh, MA, is the executive director and chief executive officer of the Long Island Association for AIDS Care, Inc., (LIAAC) in Huntington Station, New York. She received a master's degree in health education/counseling from Adelphi University and is currently a doctoral candidate in health administration and thanatology at the Union Institute.

☐ The majority of Long Island's AIDS cases are related to intravenous drug use. In fact, Nassau County ranks fifth in the nation for intravenous drug-related AIDS.[10,11]

And there's more grim reality in suburbia. Our area has a large single population and a high divorce rate. We suspect these are partial explanations for our high proportion of women with AIDS—26 percent—which is nearly three times the national average of nine percent.[12,13] Also, 10 percent of our clients acquired AIDS through heterosexual contact. Among our teenagers, drugs, the lifestyle of runaways, sexual abuse, prostitution, and even intravenous steroid use are contributing to a growing risk of HIV infection.

When LIAAC incorporated in 1986, we established that the following basic needs had to be immediately addressed. First, people felt safe seeing AIDS as a New York City problem. We needed aggressive leadership in prevention and education to disseminate reliable and accurate AIDS information. The goal was to counter the widespread apathy and denial by the public and medical professionals. Second, we needed to convince hospitals, nursing homes, adult homes, and social service agencies to face AIDS. Third, many people with AIDS needed housing. This is a problem for all Long Islanders, not just people with AIDS. Our single-family home prices are among the highest in the country, and there is a severe shortage of affordable rentals and multiple-family dwellings. Fourth, Nassau and Suffolk County governments needed to start communicating and cooperating on AIDS-related issues.

Planning for an Epidemic: LIAAC's Initial Strategies

Having identified these needs, we had to develop strategies for addressing them. Fortunately, we had assistance from the New York State Department of Health's AIDS Institute. In 1986, the AIDS Institute designated eight community service programs statewide to offer AIDS prevention education and other services. LIAAC was selected to serve Nassau and Suffolk counties.

The AIDS Institute provided basic funding for us to set up general operations after our incorporation. At the same time, we joined a consortium with the Nassau County Medical Center, the Visiting Nurses Association, and the Nassau County Department of Health to respond to The Robert Wood Johnson Foundation's (RWJF) call for proposals for a four-year demonstration grant for Nassau County.

Under the RWJF grant, the Medical Center, which has an AIDS care unit, planned a transportation project and a home-visiting physician program. The Visiting Nurses Association planned to coordinate home-care services, and LIAAC was to provide case management, prevention and education. But for us, there was an important hitch—the RWJF grant would cover only Nassau County. Fifty percent of our caseload comes from Suffolk County. If we received the grant, we would be faced with finding other ways to increase our Suffolk services so that they would match those available to Nassau clients.

LIAAC then implemented the following strategies:

First, LIAAC recruited individuals for staff, board, and volunteers who represented our entire community. We had to make it clear that we are an agency serving all Long Islanders affected by AIDS. We knew we could not succeed if we were perceived as an organization serving primarily the gay community, because 65 percent of people with AIDS on Long Island are not gay-identified.[14]

Second, we decided to expand our Hotline through volunteers. The Hotline was one of the few services we could immediately make equally available to every Long Islander, from the city line to Montauk. And given our community's fear of AIDS and their desire for anonymity, a hotline seemed to be our most viable method of communication.

Third, we implemented a comprehensive case management system for our clients. Meeting their many needs requires extensive networking between community service providers, medical institutions, and social service agencies.

Fourth, we established a free legal clinic for our clients to help solve the complex legal problems facing people with AIDS.

Fifth, we greatly expanded our support groups. We recognized the social and geographic isolation of PWAs, their families and loved ones, as well as their need to share common experiences. Support groups, each with a slightly different focus, bring these people together and help relieve their burden of isolation.

Sixth, we started a planned community relations program. This program responded to the community's almost total denial of AIDS' existence on Long Island by educating the public about the larger issues and the basic facts of HIV infection. Our program involves sending speakers to other organizations, sponsoring public events and forums, and producing public service announcements, a poster campaign, and a bimonthly newsletter.

Finally, we actively pursued partnerships with other institutions, including county governments, the religious community, and medical institutions. We needed to make clear that, while we would be offering specialized services such as a hotline, case management, support groups, a newsletter, and so forth, we all had to work together to meet such long-term needs as medical care, housing, home care, and prevention.

We knew that we were only scratching the surface in meeting the problems that AIDS was causing in our community. But we had to start somewhere. We felt that this multi-faceted approach to the demonstration project's challenge would serve the greatest number of people.

Obstacles Encountered: Expected and Unexpected

As we plunged ahead with these programs, we encountered obstacles. Some we expected. Others took us by surprise. We expected that many of our government and community leaders would be reluctant to deal with AIDS. We knew that the Island's larger problems with transportation and housing would be magnified for people with AIDS. However, even we were surprised that Nassau County avoided setting up an AIDS Commission until late 1989.

Here are four obstacles we didn't expect. We encountered continuing fear and reluctance on the part of physicians, dentists, hospitals, and long-term care institutions to both working with and planning for people with AIDS. I think we genuinely believed that these professionals and institutions, who are supposed to provide compassionate care, would come around once they were adequately educated about HIV transmission. Most have not come around, although the exceptions stand out like shining stars.

In 1987, county-wide elections resulted in a Republican majority in Nassau, but a Democratic majority in Suffolk—the first in decades. This intra-island party split, combined with the counties' completely different governmental structures, led to real problems in trying to get them to work together on AIDS. LIAAC still maintains essentially separate working relationships with both counties, although we are always looking for ways to foster bicounty efforts.

The Island's PWA population has not naturally drawn together because of AIDS. In many cities, the common background of AIDS brings about a growing spirit of belonging among diverse groups. On Long Island, people are holding onto old stereotypes, such as homophobia, racism, sexism, addictophobia, and an intolerance toward the homeless and the poor.

Finally, except for the RWJF, the Grumman Corporation, and the Veatch Foundation, we've received little support from either the business community or philanthropic foundations. Beyond small grants for specific projects, no other corporation or foundation has demonstrated much concern about AIDS on Long Island in terms of dollars. We are grateful for their recognition and praise, but we had hoped these would be matched by a financial commitment.

Hard-won Achievements

In spite of these obstacles, we've had a lot of success. Since 1986, our staff has grown to 35, and we have 350 volunteers. Together, this work force is handling a current caseload of 650 people. In all, LIAAC has helped over 1,300 people with HIV infection and 430 of their family members and loved ones.

Our Hotline is now operating 24 hours a day. From 9 a.m. to 9 p.m., Monday through Friday, trained volunteers and staff answer calls personally. We have bilingual staff available for Spanish-speaking callers. At all other times, a special computer system offers callers a variety of tapes on AIDS-related subjects. We're very proud of our Hotline. Since 1986, we've logged a total of 36,000 calls—an average of 1,000 per month.

Since its inception in 1988, our legal clinic has served over 200 clients. Its volunteer attorneys handle wills, living wills, powers of attorney, debt management, guardianship problems, and referrals in connection with discrimination and other, more complex, legal issues.

We're also very proud of our other client services. We currently run 15 support groups, which are attended by about 185 people per week. Our case managers help clients access community services and file for all benefits to which they are entitled. Each case manager is assigned from 50 to 75 clients. They're able to handle such large caseloads because of the working partnerships we've forged with Social Security, departments of social services, substance abuse treatment centers, Catholic Charities, and other not-for-profit agencies. Case managers participate in weekly rounds at the three AIDS-designated hospitals in Nassau and Suffolk.

Several strong community partnerships have formed as a result of our demonstrated excellence in case management. We work closely with the Nassau/Suffolk Health Systems Agency and have taken a leadership position in both counties' long-term planning for addressing HIV infection. The New York State AIDS Institute has substantially increased our funding, making Suffolk services comparable to those provided in Nassau. In addition, in 1988, LIAAC entered into a contract with Suffolk County to provide case management services, hotline supervision, and medical consultation.

LIAAC's effectiveness and reputation have also enabled us to act as a bridge to help close the housing gap facing our PWAs. We've brought together religious communities, social service agencies, and other not-for-profit groups toward this end. Through this networking, Long Island now has two residential supervised homes, two semi-supervised apartments, and a variety of independent living situations for PWAs. In addition, our close working relationship with Social Services helps us to maintain many PWAs in their own homes and apartments. RWJF is the only one of our grantors who has consistently recognized and supported our clients' housing needs.

RWJF and Grumman have also been important backers of our successful prevention and education efforts. The Prevention/Education Department, with the help of the minority outreach program, enabled us to deliver a total of 1,785 programs since 1986. Each month the department is responsible for 30 educational programs, two to three radio shows, two to five newspaper or magazine interviews, and two to three appearances on local cable news.

We consider our bimonthly newsletter one of our greatest accomplishments, with an annual distribution of 36,000 copies. Circulation includes clients, volunteers, families, friends, medical professionals, hospitals, social service agencies, other AIDS organizations, businesses, schools, libraries, and religious organizations. It's been highly praised for its comprehensive coverage of AIDS issues. In fact, we've received requests for copies from all over the United States as well as Europe, Asia, and Australia.

Planning for the Future: What Can We Expect?

So now, having told you what's been difficult and what we're proud of, it's time to discuss the future. As we enter the second decade of AIDS, it's instructive to look at this decade's first month to give some measure of what lies ahead.

In January, LIAAC broke its own monthly intake record with 52 new client requests and 17 family-member requests. Our average monthly intake request, until now, has been 20 to 30. On the somewhat brighter side, there were only five deaths in January. Our average had been eight to 12 deaths per month. This indicates that people with AIDS might well be living longer.

Our January client profile has not shown much change from previous months. Following is an analysis of the various modes of infection among LIAAC clients:

☐ 42%—intravenous drugs
☐ 35%—gay
☐ 10%—heterosexual
☐ 7% —bisexual
☐ 3% —transfusion-related
☐ 2% —children
☐ 1% —unknown risk.

Of this total population:

☐ 28% are minority group members
☐ 26% are women
☐ 11% come from a family in which more than one person has AIDS—usually a mother and a child.

Statistically speaking, AIDS on Long Island is likely to continue affecting the same mix of people—most of whom are disenfranchised, discriminated-against, and unempowered. LIAAC will continue to be their advocate.

Historically, publicity about the epidemic has focused on numbers and ignored the human side of AIDS. I would like to relate some stories from LIAAC's January files which reflect the human aspects of this epidemic:

☐ LIAAC supported a bill to give the right of subpoena to the Suffolk County Human Rights Commission, which would include increasing the Commission's authority to conduct investigations on discrimination-related issues involving people with AIDS. Not only was the proposal defeated, but a new proposal was put on the agenda to abolish the Human Rights Commission altogether.
☐ The VA Hospital in Northport called us in January to ask for help in bringing services to the increasing number of veterans with AIDS.
☐ LIAAC is relocating a family whose four children were physically assaulted, thrown off a school bus, and had rocks thrown through the windows of their home—all because their mother died of AIDS.
☐ We relocated a family of seven who were living in one room. The mother and one child have AIDS. Now, for the first time, each child has his or her own bed.

☐ The growth in requests for HIV-positive/asymptomatic support groups outnumbered our ability to serve this population. LIAAC decided to close these support groups and begin workshops that would accommodate larger numbers of people.

☐ We received a request from the Department of Transportation Sanitation Workers to do an educational program for 600 employees. We were asked to address their fears of picking up garbage which may contain needles.

☐ The big highlight was our collaboration with Catholic Charities to open the Island's first dental clinic for people with AIDS.

☐ We were also asked by Suffolk County to help plan a new county-run nursing home that would accept people with AIDS.

☐ However, the only county nursing home in Nassau, A. Holly Patterson, continued to refuse admission to people with AIDS.[15]

☐ As always, LIAAC was working on housing issues. In January, we sent a representative to Albany to lobby with the New York State Catholic Conference Public Policy Forum. The Forum had targeted housing for PWAs as one of its lobbying topics.

Since none of the work I've just described can be accomplished without funding, we continue our efforts to obtain financial support.

Along with directors of 11 other community service programs, I attended a private meeting with Governor Mario Cuomo to discuss services and funding. The Governor acknowledged and praised community service programs for being the front line of defense in the war against AIDS. However, the current New York State budget does not provide for any increases for AIDS community service programs. Strike one.

Extensive subcommittee meetings with the Advisory Board of the Nassau County AIDS Care Consortium have not resulted in a commitment from Nassau County to pick up any of the funding from the RWJF grant which expires on December 31, 1990. Strike two.

Our caseload will expand by 30 to 60 percent by the end of 1990. On Long Island, there cannot be a strike three.

Before leaving to come here today, I received the following letter:

Dear Ms. Barouh,

I was reading your latest edition of The LIAAC Newsletter *and decided to heed your call for a letter of support.*

I began making small donations to your organization a number of years ago for no particular reason other than a basic interest in making a contribution to a needy cause around the holidays. Although I was aware of AIDS, as many people were, from media coverage, it had yet to make a personal impact on my life. Quite frankly, I never anticipated it would.

Unfortunately, since that time a very close friend was diagnosed with the disease and has steadily become weaker and increasingly ill. I fully expect he will not survive past this year. As a result, learning to deal with AIDS head-on like this has certainly changed my life. My perception of the disease is totally different, and my concern over care for PWAs and all the research, treatment and social issues that go with that concern have been magnified beyond my wildest dreams.

Like most people who grow up in a peaceful, somewhat sheltered environment like the Long Island suburbs, I never thought I'd be touched by this crisis or almost any crisis. But here it is. Now there isn't a day that I'm not thinking about it and feeling enormous frustration, a sense of helplessness and grief that my friend must go through this.

One source of comfort has been receiving your newsletter, which has served to remind me that I am not alone. So far I have not had to utilize the many services you provide, but I'm sure some day soon I will, and it is very good to know you are there. I realize there is a great deal of expense involved in running your organization effectively, and I hope this letter along with any donations I can make will help your operation.

Although I would never wish this disease on anyone in any form, I fear it will take the general population and government officials an experience similar to mine to fully begin to feel how important your services can be. I also realize my situation is mild compared to what some people must go through.

I wish you continued success in this long battle and again thank you for the support you have already given me.

LIAAC has accomplished a great deal in four years. Some of our dreams have come true. But without stabilization of our current funding and without additional funding, LIAAC and the people we serve are in danger of losing the war against AIDS on Long Island. We have to grow as the epidemic grows. We are already beginning to lose ground.

NOTES

1. *Centers for Disease Control HIV/AIDS Surveillance Report.* Issued December 30, 1985, p. 1.

2. *AIDS Surveillance Monthly Update.* Bureau of Communicable Disease Control, New York State Department of Health, February 1986, p. 2.

3. *Centers for Disease Control HIV/AIDS Surveillance Report.* Issued December 1989, pp. 6-7.

4. "Experimental County Estimates by Age, Sex, Race, Year." Long Island Regional Planning Board, 1980-1985, Washington, D.C.: U.S. Census Bureau.

5. "Plan for a Comprehensive Response to HIV Infection and Related Diseases in Nassau and Suffolk Counties." Nassau/Suffolk Health Systems Agency, Inc., August 1988, Exhibit 1.

6. "Experimental County Estimates", op.cit.

7. "Plan for a Comprehensive Response to HIV Infection and Related Diseases in Nassau and Suffolk Counties." Nassau/Suffolk Health Systems Agency, Inc., August 1988, Exhibit 1.

8. Griggs, John, ed. "Public Policy Dimensions: AIDS." Report from Proceedings of a National Conference Sponsored by United Hospital Fund of New York and The Institute for Health Policy Studies. San Francisco, California, 16-17 January 1986.

9. Statistic from LIAAC's client profile.

10. *Centers for Disease Control HIV/AIDS Surveillance Report.* Issued December 1989, p. 9.

11. *AIDS Epidemiology Program Report.* New York State Department of Health. Albany, 31 July 1989.

12. *Centers for Disease Control HIV/AIDS Surveillance Report.* Issued December 1989, Table 6, p. 11.

13. *AIDS Epidemiology Program Report.* op.cit.

14. Statistic from LIAAC's client profile.

15. Zinman, David. "AIDS Patients Backed, State Charges Nassau Nursing Home with Bias." *Newsday* (Nassau and Suffolk editions) Long Island, New York, 6 February 1990, p. 4.

Providing Care in a County Nursing Home AIDS Unit

Shauna Dunn

Overview of AIDS in Palm Beach County, Florida

Palm Beach County is located in southeast Florida, 90 miles north of Miami. It is the largest county in Florida, with a population of approximately 850,000. Most of the population lives in a strip near the Atlantic Ocean. About 45,000 persons live in the western part of the county which is characterized by its agriculture—mainly sugar cane production.

Acquired Immune Deficiency Syndrome (AIDS) first appeared in Palm Beach County very early in the epidemic (1981). Since then, the disease has presented a pattern that differs from the general trend in this country. Compared to the United States as a whole, Palm Beach County AIDS surveillance data reveal:

☐ a smaller percentage of homosexual/bisexual males

☐ a larger percentage of intravenous drug users

☐ a larger percentage of heterosexual contact

☐ a larger percentage from other countries (especially Haiti)

☐ a larger percentage of blacks (fewer whites and Hispanics), and

☐ a larger percentage of women and children.

Development of an AIDS services network began with representatives from various organizations forming an ad hoc group to share information and the experiences they were having when clients with AIDS entered their programs. This included the Palm Beach County Public Health Unit, Hospice of Palm Beach County, Information Forum of Palm Beach County, Legal Aid Society, Palm Beach County Home and General Care Facility, and other agencies.

In 1986, this group of agencies submitted a successful proposal to The Robert Wood Johnson Foundation to develop a service demonstration project of community-based AIDS care, stressing case mangement. This resulted in the funding of the Comprehensive AIDS Program of Palm Beach County, Inc. Subsequently, other major funding has been received from federal (Health Resources and Services Administration and Centers for Disease Control), county (Children's Services Council), and private sources.

Our case management network now includes medical care, skilled nursing (long-term care facility and home care), housing, nutritional, educational, psychological, legal, and financial assistance.

The Palm Beach County Home and General Care Facility

Beginning as a "poor farm" in the 1920s, County Home has grown to a present capacity of 210 residents. It provides long-term care for indigent adults of all ages with disabling conditions requiring skilled nursing, including: dementia, spinal trauma, brain damage, mental retardation, AIDS, and others.

Shauna Dunn, RN, MS, is executive director of the Comprehensive AIDS Program of Palm Beach County, Florida. During the previous 10 years she has held clinical and administrative positions in psychiatric and chemical dependency treatment facilities and has three years of volunteer work experience in community-based AIDS organizations in Wisconsin and Florida.

Hospitalization for indigent persons is provided at private hospitals, which are reimbursed with county funds up to the amount budgeted for the fiscal year.

As early as 1982, persons with AIDS were admitted to the Home and assigned to rooms scattered among the other residents. They were kept in isolation in private rooms. As the epidemic grew, concern mounted as to how best to meet the needs of these persons and the predicted numbers of new patients with the disease.

A Designated AIDS Wing (Haney Unit)

Conceptualization of an AIDS wing was proposed as part of the service demonstration project initiative (1985-86) in keeping with the goals of quality service and cost-effectiveness.

Quality was to be improved by opening a new wing in response to the increasing number of persons with AIDS (PWAs) who were disabled and unable to remain at home. All single rooms would allow for the infection control measures thought to be necessary at the time. By clustering these younger terminal patients, a milieu would be possible that would include group therapy and social activities. Staff could receive inservice education on the latest information on AIDS care and receive added support in dealing with the issues raised by the disease. Decor would stress a homelike environment through wallpaper, soft colors, artwork, and woodwork. Practical touches include extra storage areas throughout, in particular for disposables. Special observation rooms would be located next to the nurses' station to allow for closer observation of acutely ill or newly admitted persons.

Cost effectiveness was to be achieved by reducing the number of inpatient days at acute care hospitals, which cost the county a higher per diem rate.

It was planned that the County and the private sector would jointly fund the new unit. A private grant would provide for remodeling of a wing at the County Home from a storage area into a 15-room patient care unit. The County would provide operating expenses and personnel. With the help of the county commissioner, the plan was proposed and approved by the Board of County Commissioners. However, the private funding for building renovation ($250,000) was not granted. Instead, the commissioner was successful in obtaining county funding for this expense.

On January 4, 1988, the 15-bed unit opened, named after Patrick Haney, a local AIDS educator and political activist who died from AIDS. In December 1989, 14 of the rooms were converted to semi-private, bringing the capacity of the unit to 28. Census was 20 on January 13, 1990.

Experiences/Recommendations

Negative community response to an AIDS unit has been surprisingly absent. This may be because the County Home had existed at this location for 40 years, and no new site or building was added. It was stressed that the home had already been caring for these patients for six years. Also of significance is that the neighborhood where the home is located was undergoing change at the time, from a low-income residential area to commercial and health care industry uses.

Personnel at the County Home had received in-service training on AIDS and were accustomed to caring for clients with the disease. Other patients or their families did not object significantly. Of course, residents of the County Home are indigent and are placed there because there is no family who can maintain them at home, so few other options exist for them. The greatest objection has come from the families of staff who work on the unit. With the publicity about an AIDS unit came concerns for the safety of their loved ones or the possibility of transmission to other family members. In-service training has been conducted specifically for the families of Haney Unit staff with good results. Recommendations include reaching out to families early, before a new unit is publicized.

Other personnel issues have evolved around the staff's difficulty in accepting the alternative lifestyles of their patients. Recommended is education about homosexuality, bisexuality, chemical dependence, and 12-step recovery programs. Staff who are not able to function in a therapeutic manner when these issues arise should be eliminated early on.

Recruitment of staff, especially registered nurses, was hampered by a non-competitive salary structure during approximately the first year and one-half of operation; however, with an upward adjustment in 1989, this has greatly improved.

Clinical experience has differed from what was originally expected. What was expected to be a terminally ill patient group with little time to live has not turned out to be the case. Length-of-stay varies from 10 days to years. One-third of the patients are actually discharged (including against-medical-advice discharges, administrative discharges, and scheduled discharges). Therefore, discharge planning has emerged as a major focus. Unfortunately, residents leaving the facility are faced with the same problems as our other PWAs concerning housing. Although one social worker is assigned for all the other units (190 beds), one is provided exclusively for the Haney wing. This person networks with the case managers at the Comprehensive AIDS Program to provide as smooth a transition as possible for residents.

At times, the milieu is described by one staff member as resembling a "wet shelter" where homeless chemically dependent persons find a place to stay. This has resulted in persons who, when not acutely ill, want to continue using drugs. Thus, many of the non-scheduled discharges are for bringing drugs into the unit.

Heterosexuals, IV drug and crack users, blacks, and homeless people are over-represented in the census. One-third of the patients are women. About one-third are from Western Palm Beach County, in keeping with the ratio between Coastal and Western County areas in AIDS surveillance statistics. Each person admitted must have an AIDS diagnosis and must require skilled nursing care.

Recommendations for others developing an AIDS unit are listed here:

☐ Allow the AIDS unit to develop operating procedures that differ from the other units as needed; uniformity is not practical.

☐ Provide more social service staff; for example, two staff per 28-bed unit.

☐ Seek staff who can speak Creole and Spanish or provide other means of translation.

☐ Seek staff to match the racial mix of patients.

☐ Provide daily group therapy.

☐ Offer 12-step group therapy/meetings at the facility.

☐ Organize group education to supplement one-to-one counseling.

☐ Develop an agreement between medical staff and other members of the treatment team as to clients' use of addictive substances and management of drug-seeking behavior.

☐ Provide in-service training to staff on stress mangement and mutual support techniques.

☐ Provide a staff support group if the staff desires one.

Clients have had an overall low level of functioning which is often difficult to evaluate. Illiteracy, language barriers, and multiple illnesses are complicated by a lack of baseline data, resulting in diagnostic dilemmas.

AIDS-related dementia and other neurological problems have been found in many of the clients. This can result in bizarre behavior—violent acting out, decline in self-care skills, delusional thinking, and other problems. Staff and patients can benefit from understanding these events as symptoms of disease and learning how to respond appropriately.

The physical plant has been the subject of numerous staff recommendations. In designing an AIDS unit, be sure storage areas and office areas are large enough to accommodate the amount of materials and staff needed. Office space on the unit for therapists, social services staff, and a lounge are important. Nursing has standing orders for medications to treat body lice and more isolation rooms for newly admitted patients. In numerous cases, much of the unit and many of its residents have undergone infestation treatment which could be prevented. The unit should not be too large (i.e., over 28). One bathroom per patient room is desirable.

Financially, expenses have been met by Medicaid (50 percent of patients have coverage) and County Assistance for persons who have resources above the Medicaid limit, but who cannot afford a private facility. Cost per day is $124 facility-wide, and no breakout is yet available for the Haney Unit, although it is believed to be higher there. Overall, the County Home has an annual budget of $11 million and receives reimbursements of $4 million, yielding $7 million in County support.

Volunteers have often requested to work on the unit. Their varying skills and motivations have resulted in a mixture of experiences with them. Procedures are being developed to make mandatory participation in the volunteer training program of the Comprehensive AIDS Program a criterion for acceptance at the Haney Wing. We recommend screening volunteers carefully and providing training commensurate to their duties.

One important form of volunteerism has been fundraising. Television sets and money for personal needs have been donated by groups conducting events on behalf of the unit. Once again, screening is important. Before agreeing to let the unit's name be used in conjunction with an event, we determine what the activity will be, whether the sponsors have a track record, how they intend the proceeds to be used (is it something we can do?) and, finally, how the money will be administered. A recent event netted several thousand dollars for personal needs, but a committee of the fundraisers had to approve each expenditure in advance. Since the County Home could not set up or negotiate such a system, the Comprehensive AIDS Program became the intermediary for the approval process and held the funds until disbursement.

Note: The author would like to express her appreciation to the following persons who provided her with information in developing this presentation:

Neal Moore, RN
Doris Orestis, Administrator
Molly Smith, Patient Care Coordinator
Palm Beach County Home and General Care Facility

Ron Wiewora, MD
Medical Director
AIDS Clinic, Palm Beach County Health Unit

A COMPREHENSIVE APPROACH TO
AIDS HOUSING IN A SECOND-WAVE CITY:
THE SEATTLE-KING COUNTY MODEL

Patricia L. McInturff

Programs to minimize hospitalization through provision of outpatient support services are an integral component of cost-effective and humane care for persons living with AIDS. Seattle-King County, Washington, has developed a systems approach to out-of-hospital services for people with AIDS, one of the most important elements of which is the provision of adequate housing matched to the patient's financial resources and medical needs. This review provides a brief demographic profile and history of AIDS services in our community; describes our approach to the development of services for people with AIDS with emphasis on housing programs; presents a detailed look at two unique housing programs, one in place and the other in development; and highlights the reasons behind our success and the challenges for the future.

History

King County is geographically large, with 2,134 square miles; only 16 counties in the United States are larger. Its 1.4 million residents account for about 30 percent of Washington state's population, and about 500,000 people—35 percent of the County's residents—reside in Seattle.

Seattle is often described as a second-wave city with respect to the AIDS epidemic in the United States. The epidemic curve of the disease in Seattle-King County follows that of first-wave cities—such as New York and San Francisco—by roughly three to five years. In terms of risk groups for AIDS, Seattle-King County looks a great deal like San Francisco. To date, approximately 95 percent of our cases have occurred in homosexual or bisexual men, with a small percentage in heterosexual IV-drug users. Although homosexual or bisexual men will continue to account for the majority of cases, substantial shifts in the demographics of AIDS in Seattle and King County will occur in the 1990s.

The first case of AIDS in King County was diagnosed and reported in 1982. In mid-1983, when fewer than 10 cases were recognized locally, both Seattle and King County appropriated funds to set up the AIDS Project of the Seattle-King County Department of Public Health. This early program included an AIDS assessment clinic for those at risk, a telephone hotline, an educational program, and an epidemiology program to track the epidemic and plan for future needs in housing, education, prevention, social services, medical care, and support services. In fact, we believe that Seattle and King County may have been the first local jurisdictions in the country to budget new tax-based dollars—that is, local dollars that did not pull resources from other programs—to deal with AIDS. Through January 1990, 1,194 cases of AIDS were diagnosed and reported in King County, 74 percent of the state's total.

Early in 1985, Seattle Mayor Charles Royer convened the Mayor's AIDS Task Force to identify the

Patricia L. McInturff, MPA, is director of the Regional Division of the Seattle-King County Health Department. She manages core public health programs focusing on AIDS, sexually transmitted diseases, tuberculosis, epidemiology and others for King County, the state of Washington's major urban population center.

housing needs of people with AIDS and other forms of advanced HIV infection. The Task Force included representatives from all relevant city and county governmental departments and from numerous local non-profit community organizations.

The Task Force determined that an integrated approach would be required, combining housing with health care and social services, and identified four basic housing needs:

☐ Centralized clearinghouse for coordinating housing and support services
☐ Interim housing for emergency situations
☐ Permanent housing for indigent persons with AIDS
☐ Long-term housing with on-site health care and support services.

This early work became the framework for Seattle's long-range plan for responding to the housing and support service needs of persons with AIDS and HIV disease.

By 1986, there was broad recognition among Seattle-King County policymakers and the general public about the gravity of the AIDS epidemic, and many exemplary activities were under way to serve people with AIDS. However, the many separate components had not been melded into a coordinated system. Our successful application and award of The Robert Wood Johnson Foundation funds enabled the Seattle-King County community to bring order to service delivery and to plug gaps in the system.

Central Concepts, Strategies, and Guiding Principles

Several central concepts were utilized in building Seattle-King County's continuum of AIDS care services in general and in responding to the housing needs in particular, which include: implementing a lead agency approach, providing case management services, offering a diversity of health care options, and building a strong volunteer system. Two lead agencies, one public (the Seattle-King County Department of Public Health) and one private (the Northwest AIDS Foundation), were designated to coordinate the development and implementation of community and home-based AIDS services. All other agencies and organizations were encouraged to funnel their funding proposals and coordinate their efforts through the two lead agencies, and, with few exceptions, all have done so.

First, the use of *lead agencies* facilitated program planning and implementation. This enabled the selection of the most appropriate providers to offer services through publicly supported programs; assured that appropriate standards of care were in place when programs were implemented; facilitated coordination to prevent both duplication of effort and gaps in service; and provided a mechanism to capture data needed for further program planning and evaluation.

Second, *case management services* were made available to every AIDS patient. Case managers are the backbone of the Seattle-King County care system for persons with AIDS and the glue that ties together all the elements of our larger continuum of care. At least 75 percent of persons with AIDS have had some contact with case managers; excluding contacts limited to one-time information and referral, 60 percent of persons with AIDS in Seattle and King County make active use of their case managers. The case load for each case manager has been set and generally maintained at a maximum of 40 clients.

The third central concept was the development and promotion of a *diversity of options* for persons with AIDS in the types of care available. For example, although traditional health care is emphasized, alternative approaches that do not interfere with traditional care (e.g., massage therapy, nutrition-based care) are funded and supported. This concept also is exemplified by the multifaceted approach to housing and residential long-term care. We recognize that persons with AIDS are as diverse as any other cross-section of society with respect to where they choose to obtain care, the living arrangements they prefer, and other personal issues.

The fourth key concept was to foster and support the *strong volunteer system* which has been so important in providing services. The Northwest AIDS Foundation serves as the lead agency for coordinating services by numerous volunteer agencies. These agencies include the Chicken Soup Brigade, which provides meals, chore services, and similar practical support; Shanti Seattle, which provides one-to-one emotional support; and the Seattle AIDS Support Group, which provides group support programs for patients and their families, friends, and caregivers. The use of volunteers not only saves money, but enhances the quality of life for many persons with AIDS and for the volunteers themselves.

The Seattle-King County AIDS housing program is based on a primary goal and four guiding principles. The primary goal is to provide housing services for persons in need at various stages of HIV disease, ranging from independent living to 24-hour nursing care. This continuum consists of emergency housing, independent housing, private homes and apartments, adult family homes, long-term care facilities, and hospice services. The first guiding principle is that persons with AIDS will be assisted in retaining their own personal living situation for as long as possible. Second, alternative living situations appropriate to clients' needs and desires will be made available whenever possible. Third, clients will be supported in the least restrictive setting for the maximum duration possible. The final principle is that housing will be centrally monitored and coordinated.

Program Description

As of January 1990, there were about 540 people living with AIDS in Seattle-King County. By 1993, there will be at least 2,552, and approximately 4,000 are anticipated by 1995. During 1989, 50 percent of the persons with AIDS or advanced HIV disease who resided in King County requested assistance with housing through the Northwest AIDS Foundation, the lead agency responsible for coordinating housing assistance to people with AIDS. The housing program was able to satisfy the housing needs of 85 percent of all financially eligible clients. However, most of the available housing is continually at capacity, with waiting lists.

Numerous housing options for persons with AIDS are now available in King County. Options supporting independent living include 20 Seattle Housing Authority "Section 8" certificates, which allow clients with any terminal illness to live in approved units of their choice. Currently, all 20 Section 8 certificates are being used by persons with AIDS. Clients pay approximately one-third of their income toward rent. This is the most requested housing program, with a current waiting list of 30 people.

The Seattle Housing Authority's conventional housing program, which is not specific to AIDS or any illness, enables clients to live in apartment complexes owned and managed by the Housing Authority. Selection is based on standard regulations for federally subsidized housing. To date, approximately 100 persons with AIDS have been housed through this program, which currently offers the most expedient means to house a client in a single independent unit.

Other options include four church-supported facilities, including the DeWolfe House (six units), the Multi-Faith AIDS Project (five units), Vincent House (three units), and the Payne Apartments (four units of clustered apartments), and a publicly-supported (Seattle Housing Authority) commercial housing initiative, the Cambridge Apartments (clustered apartments—nine units in 1989, expanding to 15 in 1990). Facilities offering 24-hour nursing services include Rosehedge House (six units) and the Mt. Saint

Vincent Nursing Home (two units). The Theodora Convalescent Center (units as available) is a state-licensed congregate care facility with meals and some support for activities of daily living. Housing subsidies—typically $100 to $200 per month—are provided by the Northwest AIDS Foundation and are financed by donations and gifts.

Rosehedge House

The case of Rosehedge House is illustrative of the effort behind development of each of these housing facilities. Rosehedge House was the first licensed adult family home offering 24-hour supportive care for persons with AIDS. It has facilities for six clients and opened June 20, 1988. The project was designed as a demonstration of a family home model of skilled nursing care that could be piloted in Seattle-King County to ascertain both financial feasibility and client acceptance.

The existing state law requires that an adult family home provide care to no more than four adults and that the home be owned and operated by the individual or family who permanently resides there. After several months of negotiations, the Washington State Department of Social and Health Services was willing to waive these regulations for licensure. Rosehedge House was licensed for six residents, and a nonprofit home health care agency, Community Home Health Care, was permitted to operate the facility. Community Home Health Care, with the assistance of Department of Public Health staff and funding from The Robert Wood Johnson Foundation, leased a large older house located near both Seattle's major medical centers and the neighborhood with the greatest concentration of AIDS patients. To bring the facility up to State standards, contributions and grants totaling $77,500 were raised for renovations, with the largest contribution ($36,000) coming from the Northwest AIDS Foundation. Finally, the State agreed to reimburse Community Home Health Care at an exceptional rate of pay ($229 per day).

The services provided at Rosehedge House include intravenous therapy, hospice care, volunteer support, case management services, physical therapy consultation, and several other home health services. Eligibility criteria for admission include the need for nursing care, execution of power of attorney for health care and finances, a legal will, and ability and willingness to live within a group environment.

Clients must apply and be accepted for state financial assistance and are expected to pay for their care with this monthly assistance check, retaining a small amount for personal use. Each client has a private room and access to a personal refrigerator. The house includes a shared living and dining room as well as bathing facilities. A deck addition has been added to the house to create usable outdoor space for frail residents.

During its first 18 months of operation, Rosehedge House has served a total of 55 clients, with an average of six clients on the waiting list and a mean length of stay of 60 days. Initially seen as "a place to go and die," prospective clients now understand that Rosehedge House is a community environment where they can "go and live."

This demonstration project, reimbursed through state and federal monies, is continually being evaluated by the Seattle-King County Department of Public Health. Rosehedge House not only directly serves a certain segment of the population, but is a model for smaller counties in Washington state where a larger long-term care facility will never be appropriate. Today, Rosehedge House has a waiting list of 10, and Community Home Health Care, the operating agency, has located a second facility. This second house will be purchased, rather than leased, using a combination of State Housing Trust dollars, federal monies provided under the McKinney Act, and funds from United Way of King County.

AIDS Housing of Washington

In 1988-89, a community planning group coordinated by the Seattle-King County Department of Public Health met over a six-month period to develop recommendations for both short-range and long-range approaches to the residential 24-hour care needs of persons with AIDS. The primary need identified was for a 35-bed long-term care facility. The planning group evolved into AIDS Housing of Washington. By the end of 1989, this nonprofit agency had raised $4 million of the $6 million needed for the design and construction of a 24-hour care residence for persons with AIDS.

We believe this facility will be the first of its kind in the nation. It will have 35 beds for people living with AIDS who need 24-hour care and cannot be appropriately cared for in their homes, but who do not require in-patient hospital care. The estimated daily cost will be $200, compared with an average of $800 for in-patient hospital care and $300 for 24-hour services at home. In addition, the facility will house an adult day facility, providing a supervised environment, activities, and meals for persons with AIDS who live at home and need supervision, but whose primary caregiver works or is otherwise not available during the day. Specific services that will be provided include:

☐ Housing: 35 persons with AIDS, up to 150 persons per year
☐ Hospice and Terminal Care: support and services for residents in terminal stages of AIDS
☐ 24-Hour Skilled Nursing Care
☐ Assisted Living: supervision and assistance with dressing, grooming, bathing, personal hygiene, etc.
☐ Respite Care: short-term residential care for persons with AIDS whose primary caregiver needs time off
☐ Adult Family Daycare: supervised environment, rehabilitation services, and medication management in the daytime for people with AIDS who have nocturnal care at home.

The environment at the housing facility will be as home-like as possible. Each resident will have his or her own bedroom and bath, with shared living, dining and activities rooms, a library, and a "quiet" room. Other features will include a protected courtyard, a garden, and a greenhouse. Services will be individualized. The staff will be trained to provide all levels of care to each resident, without a need for clients to move from room-to-room or wing-to-wing as the level of care changes. To the extent possible, each resident's room will become his or her home. There will be no posted visiting hours; friends and family will be continually welcomed and encouraged to visit, spend the night, and assist with care.

Table 1 summarizes the funds received as of January 1990 and illustrates the broad scope of public and community support for this project. Land for the project has been purchased, a zoning and construction permit obtained, and construction is scheduled to begin September 1990, for completion September 1991.

The State of Washington Department of Social and Health Services (DSHS) will reimburse care in the facility for people with Medicaid coverage at an exceptional rate of pay. Insurance companies have also expressed interest in reimbursing this care because of the substantial savings it offers over hospital care. The facility will be self-supporting.

Unfortunately, the sailing has not been entirely smooth. AIDS Housing of Washington has experienced some negative community reaction to this facility in the immediate neighborhood, despite overwhelmingly positive support from the media, corporations, and the general public. Although most nearby merchants support the facility, an objection to the zoning permit has been filed. Those who oppose the facility are by no means atypical, and it undoubtedly would suffer from the "not in my backyard" syndrome wherever it was located, perhaps even if it served persons with illnesses other than AIDS. However, AIDS Housing of Washington remains optimistic that fundraising and construction will proceed on schedule.

Summary and Future Challenges

In summary, our service delivery and housing programs have achieved considerable success in terms of the response of persons with AIDS, substantial reductions in the average duration of hospitalization of AIDS patients in our community, and support by government agencies at all levels, numerous philanthropic organizations, and the community at large.

We believe our success is based on several features of our program which include:

- ☐ a history of cooperation among all interested agencies and groups
- ☐ timely comprehensive planning
- ☐ lead agency approach
- ☐ centralized case management
- ☐ centralized housing coordination
- ☐ emphasis on dignity and self-esteem, and
- ☐ broad-based community support through marketing and public relations.

First is a *history of cooperation* between the Seattle-King County Department of Public Health, other government agencies and representatives, numerous philanthropic and community-based volunteer agencies, and representatives of populations at risk for AIDS. This spirit of collegiality and cooperation was initially fruitful in developing prevention and education programs and other support services that predated specific concerns about housing. Second, *timely comprehensive planning* was undertaken that involved all interested parties and agencies. The third basis for our success is our *lead agency approach,* with which came economies of scale and avoidance of both duplication of effort and gaps in service delivery, while maintaining the independence and enthusiasm of over 20 involved agencies. Fourth, the model is based on *centralized case management,* which serves, among other things, to assure that all persons with AIDS and advanced HIV infection are aware of and know how to access the options available to them. Fifth, a system was created for *centralized housing coordination* to assure the equitable distribution of housing to those most in need. Sixth, at all levels of negotiation and planning, *maintenance of dignity and self-esteem* of persons with AIDS or at risk has been the foremost concern of all participants. Finally, we have enjoyed *broad-based community support,* the direct result of carefully structured efforts to "market" our support services and housing programs to garner the needed community and political support through public forums, "working" the media, and quiet, non-confrontational diplomacy with legislators and other community leaders.

Although we have managed to serve current caseloads with the resources to date, available projections for the future are frightening, based on AIDS caseload projections in Seattle and King County. The historical experience is that 50 percent of AIDS patients will need housing, but if only current resources are available in 1995, less than one-quarter of those in need will be served. Moreover, as the proportion of cases from disadvantaged populations increases as a result of the shifting demographics of HIV infection and AIDS, the need will expand still further.

Specific future challenges include developing resources to expand the system to meet the increased numbers of cases and to provide adequate housing for AIDS patients among substance abusers, those with chronic mental illness, ethnic minority populations, women, and children.

Note: The assistance of Kurt A. Wuellner, Housing Coordinator, Northwest AIDS Foundation, and Betsy Leiberman, Executive Director, AIDS Housing of Washington, is greatly appreciated.

Table 1.

AIDS HOUSING OF WASHINGTON
COMMITTED FUNDS TO DATE

TOTAL CAMPAIGN GOAL	$5,889,629

Private Funds:

Board and Staff Donations	137,413
Individual Donations/Solicitations	121,802
Swedish Hospital Staff	1,500

Corporations and Foundations:

The Boeing Company	200,000
Catholic Archdiocese of Seattle	100,000
Jewish Community Foundation Philanthropic Fund	50,000
Northwest AIDS Foundation (Walk-a-thon) 1988	41,170
The Skinner Foundation	36,000
The Weyerhauser Foundation	30,000
The Seattle Foundation	25,000
Seafirst Foundation	25,000
Safeco	25,000
The Robert Wood Johnson Foundation	15,750
The Trainer Foundation	10,000
Nordstrom Foundation	10,000
Foundation for Group Health Co-op	10,000
US Bank	10,000

Northwest AIDS Foundation (Walk-a-thon) 1989	9,500
Titcomb Foundation	5,000
KNUA Radio/Gannett Foundation	3,500
Ben Bridge Jewelers, Inc.	3,000
Norman Archibald Charitable Foundation	2,500
Washington Mutual Foundation	2,000
Simpson Reed Fund	1,000

Public Funds:

City of Seattle Special Needs Housing Levy	1,524,724
HRSA/Residence	500,000
HRSA/Adult Day Care	450,000
Washington State Housing Trust Fund	250,000
King County Block Grant	106,739
King County Building and Modernization Fund	100,000
AIDS Omnibus Act	93,525
Non-Profit Fund	33,955

TOTAL COMMITTED TO DATE:	$3,934,078
Balance Remaining to Reach Campaign Goal	$1,955,551

QUESTIONS AND ANSWERS

The panelists answering questions included, in order of their workshop presentations:

Gail Barouh, Executive Director, Long Island Association for AIDS Care

Shauna Dunn, Executive Director, Comprehensive AIDS Program, Palm Beach County (Florida)

Patricia McInturff, Director, Regional Division, Seattle-King County Health Department

Additional comments are by: Warren Hewitt, Associate Director for Policy, Office of Minority Health, Department of Health and Human Services/Public Health Service

Judith Miller Jones, Director, National Health Policy Forum

Paul Jellinek, Senior Program Officer, The Robert Wood Johnson Foundation

Comment: (by Hewitt) Regarding housing and long-term care needs of people with AIDS, it can be worthwhile to look into properties that have liens on them for potential conversion to housing. Also, every week the *Federal Register* has a listing of unoccupied properties that could be converted for use in housing people with AIDS. Some unusual properties are available, such as the old Orlando airport.

Q: (to McInturff) What is the rationale for setting up a whole new facility for housing people with AIDS in Seattle, and what will it cost to run?

A: (by McInturff) We found that it was cheaper to build a new facility than to renovate and update an existing building. It will be run by the Sisters of Providence, and it is understood that should there be an operating loss, they will take a loss. In addition, because we are operating a small facility with special needs (35 beds), the state will be reimbursing the Sisters of Providence at an exceptional rate of pay.

Q: (to panel) What about housing for IV-drug using populations?

A: (by Barouh) On Long Island, we place non-IV-drug/alcohol using people with AIDS in independent living situations. For those who are IV-drug users, the rules must be strict. The address of the housing must remain confidential, no weapons are allowed, and no sharing of prescription drug medication. Of the PWAs who have used intravenous drugs, 85 percent go back to using some form of drugs or alcohol again.

Q: (to panel) It appears that there is more public and governmental support for PWA housing in newer areas such as the West Coast and Florida than in the Northeast, where more private and philanthropic groups exist. Does this mean that there are regional differences that must be taken into account when addressing funding?

A: (by McInturff) This may be true. On the West Coast, government and community projects tend to be the norm, and we are less likely to differentiate government-run projects from community-operated projects. We have many models for public/private partnership. Also, government is more likely to take a proactive role and get involved in needed services.

A: (by Barouh) On Long Island, Catholic Charities has been very cooperative and formed a partnership with us, in contrast to local government, which has not been nearly as responsive.

Q: (to panel) What sources of reimbursement exist for PWA housing? How is Medicaid involved?

A: (by McInturff) Negotiating an "exceptional rate of pay" ($229) was critical for Seattle's Rosehedge facility. Because Rosehedge offers the highest level of nursing home care, the expense of building and maintaining the facility is greater because of the high standards of nursing home licensure requirements.

Q: (to panel) Regarding local reactions to PWA housing, is the climate changing?

A: (by Barouh) On Long Island, local resistance is so strong that the best alternative to housing PWAs in hospitals (as is now happening) is a facility on church-owned land away from resisting groups. For example, the Catholic Church may offer an empty convent for that purpose.

A: (by Dunn) In Florida, we have a very powerful anti-tax movement whose members promote the concept that providing indigent services creates indigent people. However, a nursing home for children with AIDS has been built, and the public is reacting positively. We hope this will open the door for acceptance of community housing for adults with AIDS.

A: (not identified) A discrimination suit can be brought against facilities who refuse AIDS patients which could result in termination of their Medicaid/Medicare reimbursement eligibility.

Comment: (by Hewitt) In developing high-quality housing for people with AIDS, we need to be aware that we are dealing with a convergence of public policy considerations. For example, by the year 2020, we will need those beds for the elderly.

Comment: (by Jones) It seems we have to measure success according to the situation. For example, because Seattle was a second-wave city, not hit by AIDS until later, it had time to prepare for the coming epidemic. On the other hand, cities like New York and Washington, DC, were inundated with AIDS cases right away. So in such cities, people with AIDS are sitting in hospitals, welfare hotels, and prisons. It seems once you have a huge problem, you tend to fall farther and farther behind.

Comment: (by Jellinek) Leadership is also a key element in all these communities. When AIDS hit several years ago, the communities that had the right kinds of people in place to put together appropriate policies and programs have fared better. In addition, a city like Dallas, Texas, has a totally different political environment than Seattle, Washington. Quality of PWA care should not be a matter of geography. To provide an evenhanded response to AIDS across the country, action must come from the federal level.

New Delivery and Payment Strategies: Some Options

Human Immunodeficiency Virus Infection: Some Options for a Delivery and Payment Strategy

Donald A. Young, MD

AIDS Prevention and Services: The Private Payer's Perspective

Carl J. Schramm, PhD, JD

Putting AIDS Costs into Perspective: A Blue Cross and Blue Shield View

Steven Sieverts

☐ Questions and Answers

HUMAN IMMUNODEFICIENCY VIRUS INFECTION: SOME OPTIONS FOR A DELIVERY AND PAYMENT STRATEGY

Donald A. Young

People with human immunodeficiency virus (HIV) infection require expensive acute and long-term care services. The methods for financing and delivering care in the United States do not allow many of them to obtain needed services. Consequently, a new strategy is required to improve the care of HIV-infected people.

Three characteristics of the American health care system will influence the development of this strategy: (1) lack of universal financial protection; (2) use of acute care oriented, third-party insurance to finance care; and (3) dependence on multiple private providers to furnish services.

These characteristics, which provide the context for a discussion of delivery and payment options, are described in this paper. Then, some options for a delivery and payment strategy are presented. The relative responsibility of the government and the private sector to provide financial support is discussed first. Next, the supply of services and the role of financing in ensuring capacity are considered. Finally, options regarding entitlement, benefits, and payment methods are presented.

Characteristics of the American Health Care System

The organization, delivery, and financing of health care services in the United States differs substantially from other nations. This system, which has evolved over many years, provides advanced medical care to many Americans. Nevertheless, other needs for medical care are unmet.

Lack of Universal Financial Protection

The responsibility for financing health services in the United States is shared by the private sector and the government. Coverage of health care costs, however, is not universal. The federal government provides protection for the aged, the disabled, and people with end-stage renal disease (ESRD) through the Medicare program. The federal government also directly furnishes services to the military, their dependents, certain veterans, and American Indians. Care for some of the poor is funded jointly with the states through the Medicaid program. The federal government and the states also directly fund some providers, such as community health centers.

For many other Americans, there is a strong tradition of voluntary, private health insurance tied to the workplace. But numerous workers, the unemployed, and people with certain disabilities, such as acquired immune deficiency syndrome (AIDS), are not necessarily insured.

Third-party Insurance

The government, with some exceptions, and private organizations providing financial support generally do not deliver services directly. These organizations also generally do not directly fund the development of service capacity. Rather, a third-party health insurance mechanism is used to pay providers. The policies of third-party payers, therefore, affect the availability and use of services.

Donald A. Young, MD, has served as the executive director of the congressionally mandated Prospective Payment Assessment Commission since 1983.

People with HIV infection may be particularly affected by private health insurance policies. The practice of excluding pre-existing conditions from coverage prevents many HIV-infected individuals from acquiring insurance. In addition, the traditional insurance principle of sharing risk for very costly illnesses, such as AIDS, across large groups of people has eroded. Community-rating of large groups to determine premiums is being replaced by experience-rating of smaller groups. Consequently, a single AIDS case can adversely affect the financial welfare of an insurer or the premiums paid by members of a small group. Organizations financing care, therefore, carefully screen the individuals they enroll.

The insurance approach to financing care also requires specific identification of covered benefits. Private and government insurers have favored acute, frequently technologically intensive, services. Disease prevention, long-term care, support services, and self-administered medications are frequently excluded as benefits.

The acute care focus of health insurance is not consistent with the changing patterns of disease and disability in the United States. Health insurance serves many needs of people with acute, self-limited, or potentially curable conditions. It also serves the acute care needs of people with chronic, degenerative diseases. But neither Medicare nor private insurers provide financial protection for many of the costs associated with chronic diseases. Self-administered medications and medical and social support services needed by HIV-infected individuals frequently are not covered by traditional insurance.

Finally, private and government-sponsored insurance covers services generally accepted or proven to be safe and effective. Insurance coverage is frequently not available for new types of care where medical knowledge is uncertain. HIV infection and AIDS are a relatively new cause of disability and death. Although medical knowledge has grown rapidly, large gaps remain. New but unproven treatments may be the only hope for many people. The traditional insurance requirements of safety and efficacy, however, do not meet the needs of this new devastating disease.

Multiple Private Providers

The American public generally obtains services from many private, frequently for-profit, providers. The supply of services, however, is often determined by the availability of patient care revenues from third-party payers. Availability is, therefore, highly dependent on insurance coverage and the specific benefits eligible for payment.

At times, foundations, government grants, and other sources provide financial support to develop service capacity through demonstration and research programs. In addition, voluntary services may be provided by individuals or groups in the community. Third-party payment is necessary, however, to effectively ensure the continuing supply of services to all beneficiaries. The supply of dialysis services, for example, did not grow until the Medicare program began to pay for the care of patients with end-stage renal disease. Deficiencies in third-party payment can also reduce existing service capacity. The availability of sophisticated trauma care is currently threatened by the large number of trauma patients without insurance coverage.

A single provider rarely furnishes all the services required to meet the needs of individuals with complex problems such as AIDS. The services furnished by multiple community-based providers are infrequently coordinated. Patients, therefore, may have difficulty identifying and obtaining access to services. In addition, insurance coverage is not available for some services. Therefore, people with complex or chronic conditions usually lack continuing access to comprehensive care. This may result in overuse as well as underuse of certain services.

Options for a Payment and Delivery Strategy

Three groups of policy options—relating to financing, service capacity, and scope of services delivery—to improve the care of people with HIV infection are discussed below. The options are broad, and additional decisions are necessary for a fully developed strategy. In many cases, an intermediate choice between two options is possible. The preferred option in one category may affect the choice in another. Therefore, the order in which the options are presented and discussed may influence the development of the strategy.

Finally, the options focus on the financing and delivery of services to individuals. Options related to the identification of cases and the prevention and control of the AIDS epidemic from a public health perspective are not explicitly presented.

The Source of Financial Support

Four options concerning the source of financial support are discussed in this section. In considering these options, the high cost of care for people with HIV infection must be recognized. The American public, through government or private mechanisms, may not be willing to commit all the financial support necessary for this care. Needs such as those of the uninsured population, long-term care services, and comprehensive care for other chronic conditions are likely to compete vigorously for available resources.

Option 1. Federal Government Support—The federal government could assume full responsibility for the financial support of patients with HIV infection. The need to identify, treat, and control this major public health problem to protect the welfare of all Americans supports this choice. Further, the high costs of care and the rapid advances in medical knowledge may limit the ability of many private or state and local government entities to support state-of-the-art, comprehensive care. Federal government support is also most likely to ensure equal treatment for all Americans.

The federal government could expand the Medicare program, as it did with end-stage renal disease, to include HIV-infected people. Financing could be through the Medicare payroll tax or general revenues. The waiting period for Medicare eligibility under disability rules could also be reduced or eliminated. This approach, however, may not cover the costs of treating HIV infection prior to the development of AIDS.

Alternatively, the Medicaid program could be expanded to finance comprehensive benefits for HIV-infected people. A new program with a dedicated tax is also possible.

Option 2. State and Local Support—Many states and communities currently support the care of some AIDS patients through Medicaid or other programs. This option requires state and local governments to greatly expand this effort. The rationale for this choice is based partly on the state's responsibility for maintaining public health. Further, before the enactment of Medicare and Medicaid, state and local governments provided much of the financial support for services to individuals lacking the financial means to obtain care.

State and local governments may be able to develop more innovative and creative means to furnish care consistent with local needs and circumstances. New sources of revenue, presumably taxes, would be necessary, however, for state or local governments to assume this responsibility. In many areas, the public is likely to oppose tax increases. As a result, the amount of financial support and service capability may vary widely across states and communities.

Option 3. Private Sector Support—Private insurance coverage currently finances some of the care furnished AIDS patients. Many individuals, however, are not covered because they are unemployed, disabled, or do not have the means to purchase insurance. The relationship of HIV infection to drug abuse further limits employment-based insurance as a general strategy. Once an individual is known to be infected, preexisting condition exclusions prevent the purchase of individual policies. Many insurance policies also have lifetime spending limits. In addition, a full array of benefits, especially support services and medications, are rarely covered.

Further, the large number of insurance plans with relatively few enrollees limits the ability of many plans to share the financial risk associated with the care of an AIDS patient.

Major changes in the role and responsibility of private insurance are necessary to provide broader financial support for the care of HIV-infected people. The government could mandate coverage through the workplace. Risk-sharing arrangements or re-insurance pools could be established. Nevertheless, large groups of individuals would remain uninsured. Therefore, a strategy relying entirely on private insurance is not likely to be successful.

Option 4. Mixed Government and Private Support—The joint responsibility of the private sector and government to finance health care could be continued by expanding the current level of government and private insurance. There are likely to be ongoing disputes, however, regarding relative roles and responsibilities among business, private insurers, and the government. Consequently, gaps in coverage may occur.

Alternatively, federal, state, and local governments could share responsibility, using direct funding rather than insurance. For example, the federal government could provide grants to states or communities for a portion of the costs of care. This option is considered further in the next section.

Discussion—Financial support from the federal government for the care of HIV-infected individuals may be the most comprehensive approach. Budget and political considerations, however, may limit the acceptance of a comprehensive strategy.

Shared responsibility for financing of services is consistent with current methods of financing health care. This strategy would also face budget and political obstacles. Since financial responsibility would be shared by many groups, however, these obstacles may be overcome.

Relying solely on state and local financing or private insurance would be a departure from current approaches, which include the federal government as a major contributor to health care financing. These strategies also might result in significant gaps in coverage.

Developing and Maintaining Service Capacity

Financial support for the care of HIV-infected people will increase the supply of services. The methods for funding service capacity, however, may influence the overall supply as well as the distribution of specific services. Two options for developing and maintaining service capacity are discussed.

Option 1. Direct Funding of Service Supply—This strategy requires the government or other entities to furnish services or to fund the supply of services directly. This approach would be a major departure from current methods of financing the supply of services for most Americans. A federal program of grants to the states could provide the financial support to develop service capacity and ensure access to care. The costs of the program could be assumed by the federal government. Alternatively, the states could share in the costs.

The federal government generally has not provided direct funding to ensure service delivery. However, there are exceptions. For many years the government supported hospital construction through the Hill-Burton program. The government has also provided direct financial support through the states for community health centers and other services.

State and local governments have assumed more responsibility than the federal government for direct funding and delivery of service. Nevertheless, most health care is not directly furnished by state and local governments.

Health care services are also infrequently furnished or paid for directly by private employers. Most commonly, a third party has paid a provider for the care delivered. The growth of employer self-insurance, capitated payment, HMOs, and managed care plans, however, is blurring this distinction.

As with the government, in the private sector there are exceptions to the general pattern of third-party insurance. Many companies now offer on-site services for the care of occupation-related conditions, as well as general medical services. Some private companies, for example the Southern Pacific Railroad, have provided care directly to their employees.

Option 2. Fund the Supply of Services from Patient Care Revenues—This option follows the current approach of relying on revenues from services furnished to develop service capacity. These revenues generally come from the patient or third-party insurers representing employees and the government. State and local governments also supplement the budgets of teaching and public hospitals and community health centers. The supply of services is, therefore, directly related to the availability of patient care revenues. Consequently, the capacity to provide care to all who need it requires financial support for each patient. Further, coverage of chronic care services would be required.

Discussion—The direct delivery of services by federal, state, or local governments to HIV-infected individuals would ensure service capacity. There are precedents for this approach, although it is a departure from prevailing methods. This option, however, is likely to be opposed by physicians and other providers, who would prefer a patient revenue strategy.

Alternatively, federal, state, and local governments could provide direct funding for delivery of services by private providers. People with HIV infection, however, require many services from both traditional and nontraditional providers. A direct funding mechanism that covers required services would be difficult to design and implement. It is likely that gaps in coverage would remain.

A strategy relying on patient care revenues could ensure service supply and capacity. To be successful, however, universal financial protection is necessary. In addition, all the services required by HIV-infected individuals would have to be covered.

Entitlement, Benefit, and Payment Strategies

The choice of options in this section will determine the scope of the payment and delivery strategy.

Entitlement Options

The individuals who are entitled to services under a delivery and payment strategy must be clearly specified. Entitlement can be determined by characteristics of the patient, the disease, or the treatment required. It can also be determined by an individual's age, functional status, or financial status. All of these approaches are used by the Medicare or Medicaid programs for specific groups of people.

One option is to entitle all individuals with HIV infection. Alternatively, AIDS or AIDS-related conditions could be precisely defined and determine entitlement. A third option could entitle individuals with HIV infection to a limited number of benefits, such as self-administered drugs, while people with AIDS could be entitled to full benefits. Financial status could be an additional requirement for entitlement, as it is in the Medicaid program. Many variations on these options can be considered.

Entitlement policies are likely to be complicated by rapidly expanding knowledge regarding HIV infection. For example, new information has demonstrated the value of early therapeutic intervention. Since the treatment is costly, this finding may support entitlement when HIV infection is documented.

Individuals with HIV infection are likely to require care for services unrelated to their infection. Policymakers also must decide if entitlement to HIV-related services carries with it entitlement to other services.

Benefit Options

A benefit package could include comprehensive acute and long-term care services or a limited number of the most necessary services. Different benefit packages could be designed based on the stage of the disease or other characteristics of HIV infection.

Traditional health insurance coverage is biased in favor of acute medical care and institutional services. Home health and nursing facility benefits frequently require a skilled level of care. Self-administered medications like azidothymidine (AZT) and pentamidine are frequently excluded. Counseling, support services, and new treatments are also excluded. Many of the services not covered by traditional insurance are essential to a comprehensive care strategy. They also add to its cost. Consequently, trade-offs may be necessary among benefit options.

The demand for services will increase as the financing and supply grows. Therefore, benefit design should also consider options to control utilization. Third-party payers, however, have experienced limited success in the utilization review of noninstitutional services. Determining the appropriate use of many social and support services is likely to be especially difficult.

Benefit options can be linked to payment options. The Medicare hospice benefit is an example of this strategy. A broad benefit package was developed with a preset payment amount. Providers can select medical and support services based on the needs of individual cases. Providers, however, face a strong incentive to control the use of services, since the total payment is fixed. The payment method, therefore, reduces the need to identify each benefit. The need for utilization review is also reduced.

Payment Methods and Amounts

There are two broad approaches for a payment strategy: one is to pay providers directly for services furnished; the alternative is to use a third-party insurance mechanism to compensate providers.

A strategy of direct payment to providers was considered in the discussion of services supply. A direct-payment option for services to HIV-infected people would depart from current practices. Further, direct payment would be complicated to administer. This approach, however, could rapidly improve access to care for many people.

Direct payment could also be made to an organization functioning as a case manager. This option is similar to third-party insurance and is considered in the next section.

The options for a third-party payment method include fee-for-service, cost-reimbursement, prospectively set rates for a group of services, and capitation or managed care. Funding sources, however, are not likely to support fee-for-service or cost-reimbursement methods which lack effective controls on utilization and overall costs.

An alternative payment method uses financial incentives to control the use of services. These incentives include setting a specific payment amount in advance for a group of services. Providers thus would have an incentive to control their services. The Medicare program uses this approach for payment of ESRD, hospice, and inpatient hospital services.

The same financial incentive has led Medicare and private payers to encourage enrollment in health maintenance organizations and other managed care programs. This payment strategy is intended to allow providers flexibility in matching specific services to patient needs while controlling the aggregate payment.

A single payment amount could be made to a case manager to cover all HIV-related services. Alternatively, a case manager could be used for core services. Alternative methods would be used to pay for other services. This approach would be difficult to design and administer. However, it would allow flexibility in meeting diverse patient needs. It would also reduce other problems related to determining benefits and ensuring appropriate utilization.

The final payment option concerns beneficiary cost-sharing requirements. Traditional insurance plans require some beneficiary cost-sharing through deductibles and copayments for specific services.

The payment and delivery strategy could be developed without a beneficiary cost-sharing requirement. Alternatively, a cost-sharing policy could be developed to provide incentives for the beneficiary to use services appropriately or simply to reduce the costs of the organization responsible for financing the strategy. If a cost-sharing policy is preferred, a maximum limit on beneficiary liability should also be considered.

The cost-sharing strategy may influence access to care. Therefore, the details of the policy should be considered after the payment and delivery strategy is more fully developed.

Discussion

Policy decisions regarding entitlement, benefits, and payment methods will determine the scope of coverage and mix of services available to HIV-infected people. These decisions, therefore, will determine the cost of the payment and delivery strategy. At some point, cost concerns may be a dominant factor in the development of the strategy. If so, difficult choices and tradeoffs may be necessary among the entitlement, benefit, and payment options.

Conclusion

HIV-infected people require expensive acute and chronic care services. Many of these people, however, are not receiving needed services. These barriers to care for individuals with HIV infection are due in large part to the current methods for financing care in the United States. The current shared government and private responsibility for financing of services leaves many individuals without financial protection.

Federal, state, and local government, as well as the private sector, could assume greater responsibility for financing care. A federal government strategy may be the most comprehensive. Budget and other concerns, however, may favor a shared responsibility.

The supply of services in the United States is frequently determined by the availability of health insurance and third-party payment. Patient care revenues are, therefore, an important incentive for developing service capacity. A payment and delivery strategy can continue to rely on third-party payment to determine the supply of services. Alternatively, the organizations responsible for financing care could directly furnish services or directly fund the supply of services. The American public, however, has traditionally favored a third-party insurance approach.

The scope and cost of a payment and delivery strategy will be determined by the choice of entitlement, benefit, and payment options. The specific individuals entitled to services have to be identified. Entitlement can be based on stage of infection, requirements for specific services, individual financial status, or other factors.

The benefits to be covered by the strategy also have to be specified. Third-party insurance, both government and private, has focused on acute medical care services. Self-administered drugs, long-term care, and support services frequently are not covered. To be effective in serving people with AIDS, however, a payment and delivery strategy will have to consider covering these services.

Finally, the methods and amounts of payment will influence access to care. Effective utilization controls are likely to be required for any strategy.

Improvements in the delivery of services to people with HIV infection will be expensive. A payment and delivery strategy will likely have to compete with other needs for resources.

AIDS PREVENTION AND SERVICES: THE PRIVATE PAYER'S PERSPECTIVE

Carl J. Schramm

Introduction

It is often said that AIDS points to the many problems in our health care delivery and financing system, and indeed, the difficulties in securing appropriate services for people with AIDS are reflective of generic problems that exist in the system. Among them are:

☐ the failure of Medicaid to cover the poor, with the program presently covering only about 40 percent of those living in poverty

☐ inadequate government reimbursement to hospitals and physicians which has created a serious disincentive to provider participation in the Medicaid program

☐ the lack of employer-sponsored coverage for many employed people

☐ the absence of high-risk pools for medically uninsurable people for those who are able to afford, but unable to obtain, coverage. At present, only 18 states have such pools, and many of these have had limited success.

☐ the lack of good chronic care models, not only in regard to caring for people with AIDS, but also for an aging population. Long-term care, home health, and hospice services are often unavailable or inadequate.

☐ the lack of adequate resources for substance abuse treatment and prevention.

Because AIDS is a communicable disease, a committed and strong public sector role is required. As the growth in the spread of AIDS continues disproportionately to affect populations that tend to be poor and sometimes unemployed, the need for a public sector solution to ensure access to care for the poor is essential.

The Role of the Insurer

AIDS has had a significant impact on commercial health and life insurers, who paid out approximately $500 million in AIDS-related claims in 1988. Although claims have not reached the magnitude that earlier forecasters feared, significant annual increases in claims are expected. As a substantial payer of the medical care bill for AIDS patients, the insurer has every reason to facilitate the delivery of the most appropriate, high quality, and cost-effective care.

Against the current of a provider-driven delivery system that overemphasizes acute care, insurers have sought to develop alternative methods of managing patients with serious illnesses, and most recently have begun to do so for their insureds living with AIDS. Case management, though by no means new, is being used very successfully in the management of AIDS cases, with demonstrated improvements in both costs and quality of care. With such plans, insured AIDS patients are able to receive the custodial and non-traditional support services often not covered by conventional health insurance plans, and the insured are

Carl Schramm, PhD, JD, is president of the Health Insurance Association of America (HIAA), the trade association for the nation's commercial health insurance companies. The HIAA represents some 320 health insurance companies, which provide coverage for about 95 million people.

allowed involvement in decisions about their care. Case management approaches to AIDS are essential to ensure a continuum of care throughout the course of the individual's illness.

Such innovations are also being found in the design of life insurance products. Several companies have introduced "living benefits," whereby terminally ill policyholders can collect their death benefit while living, with the funds being used at their own discretion.

In addition to meeting contractual obligations to policyholders with AIDS, the insurance industry continues to be a large corporate donor to AIDS education, prevention, and research activities. Just last year, the HIAA and the American Council of Life Insurance (ACLI) launched a three-year, $16 million grantmaking program for AIDS projects, funded by the association's member companies. A portion of these funds is being awarded by the HIAA/ACLI to support community-based AIDS service organizations in areas of low incidence or where few services are available. With contributions expected to reach $30 million by 1991, the insurance industry remains the largest corporate donor for AIDS, and the nation's third largest donor, following The Robert Wood Johnson Foundation and the government.

Increasing Access to Care for PWAs

Probably no other disease so urgently points to the need for comprehensive solutions that serve to ensure access to health care than AIDS. Programs targeted specifically to AIDS may be necessary for the short term, yet are likely to become vulnerable to an increasingly complacent public, as well as to competing demands upon limited health care resources. Rather, a renewed and strengthened commitment from the public sector to provide for the poor and continued protection through the private sector are required to meet the financing challenges posed by the AIDS epidemic.

Significant reforms in our health care financing system are well under way at the federal level and in the states. The HIAA has been vigorously developing and advancing its own four-point proposal for universal coverage, which calls upon the resources of both the public and private sectors. Specifically, our proposal calls for the following:

1. Medicaid coverage should be available to all people with incomes below the federal poverty level, regardless of family structure, age, or disability status. Priority should be given to primary care and preventive services. A Medicaid buy-in program should be available that provides a limited package of primary, preventive, and related ambulatory care to be purchased by individuals and families with incomes above poverty but below 150 percent of the federal poverty level.
2. Insurers should be allowed to offer more affordable coverage, including prototype plans, through the extension of ERISA preemption of state-mandated benefits to plans that insure employees.
3. Coverage must be made available to all Americans, including uninsurable employer groups and uninsurable individuals. Small employer groups would be able to purchase and maintain affordable coverage even if one or more of their employees is high risk. Individuals who are ineligible for employer coverage, Medicare, or Medicaid should have coverage available through a qualified state pool for medically uninsurable individuals.
4. Small businesses should be given a greater incentive to provide coverage, by allowing a 100 percent federal tax deduction to the self-employed owner for their own health insurance protection, if they provide equivalent coverage to their employees.

How we ultimately achieve universal coverage will not be determined merely by implementing the successful plan. Rather, ensuring access to care will depend heavily on having sufficient resources available. Until and unless we are successful at containing expenditures for acute care, it will be unlikely that ample resources will be available to provide primary care for those presently lacking such access, as well as developing the much needed alternatives.

Putting AIDS Costs into Perspective: A Blue Cross and Blue Shield View

Steven Sieverts

Introduction

A dread disease has become epidemic in the United States of America. More accurately, it is not a single disease; it is a group of related illnesses characterized by the weakening and breakdown of the body's normal biological defense mechanisms. That breakdown leads to the uncontrolled spread of pathology to specific organs of the body: the lungs, the skin, the brain, and others. Frequently, the result is death.

This disease is singularly and properly feared by the American public. Nevertheless, a great many Americans continue to practice personal behavior that is known to increase greatly the likelihood of becoming a victim. While not without measurable effects, even a substantial educational effort in the schools and the media—with recent new emphasis from the government—has not succeeded in persuading a great many people to abandon personal practices which are known to increase the risk of contracting this disease.

This disease is very unevenly distributed in this country. The death rates vary widely among the states and among racial and ethnic groups. Even after age-adjusting the statistics, the rates in the highest states are well over double the lowest. Rates among the poor are higher than among the middle-class, and rates among blacks are higher than among whites. Half a dozen states account for half of the reported cases. This year, about a million Americans will be diagnosed as having this feared disease. Within five years, about 600 thousand of them will have died. These are truly frightening numbers!

Not surprisingly, caring for persons who are struck by this group of diseases is very costly. Current estimates are that nearly $21 billion was expended during 1985 to care for affected persons. That amount has risen annually at double-digit percentage rates.[1] Our estimate for 1989 puts it at about $35 billion.

Quite obviously, I hope, I am *not* talking about acquired immune deficiency syndrome (AIDS). I've been discussing cancer.

Cancer is a disease, a group of diseases, that has plagued mankind for millennia. In the current era, both the incidence of cancer and cancer death rates are on the rise. During 1930, the age-adjusted death rate from cancer was 143 per 100,000 Americans. In 1950, it had risen to 158 deaths per 100,000. By 1986 it had gone up to 171 deaths per 100,000—and it was still rising. *Yet we take cancer largely for granted.* We've gotten used to it, to spending many billions to treat its victims and billions more in medical research. No one is indifferent to the tragedy of cancer, but no one is predicting that cancer care will swamp the American health care system or bankrupt American health care financing either.

A Comparison of AIDS and Cancer Statistics

Let's put those cancer statistics into perspective by comparing them to AIDS statistics.

In 1989, the federal Centers for Disease Control (CDC) counted 35,238 new cases of AIDS. The final total will be somewhat higher.[2] That is tragically many people; compounding the tragedy is the relative

Since 1985, Steven Sieverts has served as vice president of health care finance with Blue Cross and Blue Shield of the National Capital Area in Washington, DC.

youth of most AIDS patients. Compare that, however, to the American Cancer Society's (ACS) estimate of more than a million new cases of cancer, nearly 30 times more. For 1989, the CDC has reported under 15,000 AIDS deaths; the ACS estimates over half a million cancer deaths; again, about a thirty-fold difference. The $23 or so billion spent on medical care for cancer patients compares to under $2 billion for AIDS patients in 1987.[3] The $35 billion we estimate for cancer care in 1989 is probably more than ten times the AIDS and HIV-disease care costs.

Yet one hears predictions of utter societal disaster because of the crushing medical care cost burden of AIDS. Those predictions have included alarms about impending crises due to inadequate hospital beds, physicians, and nurses. Some have foreseen the collapse of America's health care financing systems under the load of paying for the care of persons with AIDS. And, perhaps understandably, we are seeing some misguided, inhumane, and just plain wrong responses from a few public officials, health care providers, and, sad to say, health insurers, too, both in the United States and abroad, based on this perception of an imminent AIDS-induced economic and medical care disaster.

The Changing Population of AIDS and HIV Patients

There will continue to be increases in AIDS cases in the United States for years to come. Even if there were no new HIV infections at all (we are far from achieving that), the present large population of infected individuals assures that. But just how large will the increase be? The federal government estimated three years ago that there were between a million and a million and a half people in that population. Experts even today are divided as to whether the true number is well below or well above that broad estimate. A million HIV-infected people would be about 40 persons per 10,000, across all ages and across the whole country.

The U.S. military continues to do HIV-antibody screening on active-duty personnel and on new recruits. It repeatedly finds that only about 15 persons per 10,000 are infected. This population is predominantly relatively young and male, with an over-representation of blacks and Hispanics. These are the very groups in the population that are at the highest risks of HIV infection. Therefore, I suspect that even the lower-bound estimate of a million infected people may be too high. But we really don't know for sure. The New York City Department of Health last year reduced its estimate of the infected population by half, for apparently sound reasons.

What does seem clear is that the HIV-infected population is changing its nature, with new cases increasingly being predominantly among persons in a few low-income urban communities and principally black and Hispanic. The most distressing increase is to be found in the numerically small but especially tragic incidence of HIV infection and AIDS among newborns, related to the social breakdown found in some urban slums where drug abuse, poverty, and family disintegration are epidemic.

We often hear that the incidence of new cases is doubling each year. Not any longer:

1983: 2,852 cases of AIDS
1984: 5,762 cases of AIDS
1985: 10,598 cases of AIDS
1986: 16,646 cases of AIDS
1987: 22,680 cases of AIDS
1988: 32,196 cases of AIDS
1989: 35,238 cases of AIDS

Those certainly are somewhat understated, and they surely aren't happy numbers, but they do show a gradual flattening of the growth curve. And with what is now known about the length of the latent period of HIV infection before AIDS appears, the numbers do not seem consistent with estimates of a million or more HIV-infected Americans.

As to geographic distribution, 22 percent of 1989's new cases were in greater New York (including northeastern New Jersey), and 12 percent were in San Francisco and Los Angeles. Put differently, metropolitan areas with about a tenth of the nation's population reported more than a third of the nation's AIDS cases last year. A third of the 50 states had fewer than 100 AIDS cases recorded in 1989, and a sixth had less than 50. There is good reason to believe that most of those stricken people became infected somewhere other than in those states, returning home for their terminal illnesses. In other words, it is reasonable to say that for most of this country, the AIDS epidemic is not quantitatively significant at this time.[2] In a few metropolitan areas, or more precisely, in a limited number of local jurisdictions, AIDS looms large as a public health problem and a medical care crisis, but not in most of the nation. This by no means is a declaration that the HIV epidemic is a minor phenomenon. Quite the contrary, it's a statement that it's a problem that America has the capacity and the resources to deal with appropriately.

The Costs of Caring for AIDS Patients

How much does it cost to provide health care for a person with AIDS? There is no single answer to that question, for three reasons:

First, as is well-known, AIDS is not a single disease in and of itself. It is a number of different illnesses that may arise in an individual whose natural immune response system has been damaged by HIV infection. The health care that a person with AIDS requires depends on what specific illnesses the individual contracts, ranging from *Pneumocystis carinii* pneumonia to Kaposi's sarcoma, and from tuberculosis to candidiasis to dementia and wasting. How much of what kinds of health services are needed depends on which illnesses, in what combination, the individual comes down with. The range, expressed as lifetime costs, is from just a few thousand dollars for some who die rather quickly to hundreds of thousands of dollars for a very few who may require repeated hospitalizations, large amounts of expensive medication, and long-term nursing care.

Second, treatments for AIDS patients have evolved rapidly in these early years and now typically involve significantly fewer hospital days on average. Some of our health maintenance organizations, and most particularly some of the Kaiser Permanente health plans, have shown that case management often results in better care at less cost. Our experience at Blue Cross and Blue Shield of the National Capital Area confirms this. Simultaneously, survival times have increased, which extends the need for nursing care and drug therapy. Some of the more encouraging current clinical findings seem to show that certain drugs, if they are administered early, may prolong the remaining life expectancy of patients dramatically. Physical fitness of the HIV-infected person and, in particular, an absence of other sexually transmitted diseases serve to ward off opportunistic infections. Proper nutrition apparently helps significantly in holding down the frequency and duration of AIDS opportunistic infections. The consequence seems to be substantially lower costs per month for health care for AIDS patients, but substantially more months during which to incur them.[4]

Third, most AIDS cases to date have been homosexual men, neither very young nor very old, living in urban areas, largely in or near neighborhoods which support substantial gay communities. Those communities have responded remarkably with formal and informal networks of volunteers, health care professionals, and health care institutions to serve AIDS patients, often at little or no charge. Moreover, especially with respect to young male homosexual adults, the families of AIDS patients have been encouraged and supported by those networks to play active roles. However, the rapid growth of persons with AIDS as a direct or indirect consequence of drug use means that relatively more and more of them will neither feel comfortable with nor will seek the help of the voluntary structures set up by and for homosexuals, and the gay-oriented support networks may not feel motivated to put equivalent effort into drug abusers with AIDS. Without any equivalent of the strong base of volunteering that heratteningly undergirds the gay community's efforts, the largely "underclass" AIDS sufferers, including most women and infants with AIDS, must rely on services from persons and facilities that expect (or at least hope) to get paid or subsidized.

How much, then, does an AIDS patient cost to care for in the United States? The estimates in the literature vary enormously. A recent study by the federal government is an attempt to pull together and make sense out of them. That study's estimate of $57,000 as the current lifetime cost seems reasonable.[5]

That study also estimated the 1988 incidence of newly diagnosed AIDS cases at 38,000 (higher by about a sixth than the CDC estimate), which works out to nearly $2.2 billion for their lifetime costs, spread over several years.

The costs of caring for AIDS patients just in 1988 were also about $2.2 billion. That can be compared to total U.S. spending from all sources, for all diseases, for all personal health care services in 1988 which was almost half a trillion dollars. AIDS therefore represented less than one-half of one percent of what this country spent for health care that year.

The federal study estimates 1991 AIDS expenditures at $4.5 billion. By then, total national health care expenditures will probably be about $650 billion, so AIDS care expenditures will have climbed to about three-fourths of one percent of the total.

One-half of one percent, three-fourths of one percent two years from now—those are obviously manageable numbers. Paying for AIDS care in the United States, with by far the highest incidence and prevalence of the disease among the industrialized nations, really shouldn't be an issue in terms of national public policy, if the concern is economic capacity to bear the burden. During the next three years, making moderate assumptions about inflation rates, U.S. spending for health care will go up more than $150 billion per year. Increases in AIDS spending will represent less than 1.5 percent of that growth.

Insurance for AIDS Care

Paying for health care services for most persons with AIDS is unquestionably the responsibility of the private sector health service plans in which such persons are enrolled. The vast majority of the HIV-infected population, other than those whose infection is related to drug abuse, have been employed people who have health insurance. It is very rare for health insurance contracts to exclude any specific disease categories as such. Only with respect to mental health services (and sometimes to obstetrical care, a non-disease category of service) does one find disease-specific differentiation in benefits in an appreciable proportion of contracts in this country. There were a few efforts by some employers and unions to exclude from benefits any AIDS-related services, but they seem not to have taken hold.

AIDS-related services are therefore usually covered no differently, with no different limitations or exclusions, than are cancer-related, stroke-related, or any other category of health care services.

Can insurance plans "afford" to cover persons with AIDS? Obviously, an American plan that enrolled a cross-section of the U.S. population would be paying out below one percent of its resources for AIDS-related care. But the plans do not, in fact, enroll random cross-sections. The voluntary non-profit sector—predominantly Blue Cross and Blue Shield organizations—and the health maintenance organizations are regional in nature. Some regions have a far higher prevalence of AIDS than others, and high-risk persons are more common in some plans than others.

Within each region, the plans enroll mainly persons covered through employer-sponsored health benefit programs, plus a relatively small number of persons who are not covered by group programs. Let us look at the experience of one such plan: Blue Cross and Blue Shield of the National Capital Area, serving the Washington, DC, region. We have reliable data on AIDS for somewhat less than half of that organization's membership—for about 450,000 subscribers, excluding those who are also Medicare beneficiaries (not employed and age 65 and older), as well as those enrolled in the national Blue Cross and Blue Shield Federal Employee Program.

The Difficulties of Counting AIDS Patients

Before proceeding, a word is in order about the difficulty of discovering AIDS cases in a claims data base. Generally speaking, persons with AIDS are not hospitalized and do not get other covered services directly because of their AIDS.

Information about primary diagnosis is obtained from the provider on each claim for institutional and professional services, but those diagnoses relate to the opportunistic infections and malignancies that afflict persons with AIDS. There wasn't even an ICD-9 code for AIDS until 1987. (ICD-9 codes refer to the International Classification of Diseases—9th Revision disease coding system, used for indexing hospital records.) None of these diseases is exclusively AIDS-related; persons who are not HIV-infected also get them. What that means is that the claims data base has to be searched intensively for cases with the diagnoses that have some likelihood of being AIDS-related. Those cases then have to be studied individually, in terms of their total claims histories over time, to ascertain which of them display patterns typical of AIDS. We are prohibited from doing direct inquiries to the providers or the subscribers about whether a particular patient has AIDS.

That search process turned up about 214 cases, out of the 450,000 BC-BS enrollees, during 1985, 1986, 1987, and 1988. Those 214 cases accounted for estimated benefits costs as follows:

$ 500,000 in 1985
$2,000,000 in 1986
$3,000,000 in 1987
$4,200,000 in 1988

The Washington, DC, metropolitan area ranks fifth in the nation in the incidence and prevalence of AIDS. Its population is over 3.3 million; just about three million are under age 65. During 1985, 1986, 1987, and 1988, there were about 2,010 reported AIDS cases, virtually all under age 65. Among the 450,000 Blue Cross and Blue Shield subscribers under age 65 in the data base, we believe we identified about 11 percent of the region's AIDS cases, probably well over 15 percent of the persons with AIDS who have health insurance.

In relation to the plan's benefit expenditures for the 450,000 subscribers, the costs of the 214 AIDS cases represented a growing fraction from about one-fifth of one percent to about nine-tenths of one percent over the four years. Blue Cross and Blue Shield of the National Capital Area, while it is deeply concerned about the epidemic's human costs, is not at all alarmed at this time about those numbers and those trends.

Are these numbers deflated because a sizable number of persons with AIDS lost their jobs and thus their coverage? Perhaps, although we have not been able to confirm this from our records. It does appear that the large majority of those whose coverage with our plan ended did so at death.

Questions and Answers About AIDS and Insurance

This is not at all to imply that there are not issues to be faced regarding health insurance and AIDS. This paper will conclude by discussing five common questions about AIDS and insurance.

1. *Should applicants for health insurance be required to submit to HIV antibody testing?* The U.S. commercial health insurance industry has said yes.[6] The voluntary non-profit plans generally say no.[4] There is surely a potential for expensive adverse selection if uninsured persons who are HIV-infected can apply for and obtain health insurance. Finding ways to keep them out of the insurance pool is therefore tempting. Requiring the HIV antibody test, however, creates two major problems.

First, the incidence of HIV infection is so low—far below one percent of the population—that testing will produce very few positive test results, proportionately speaking. If 1,000 tests produce only one or two positive findings, up to $100,000 will have been spent to uncover and deal with those cases (which could actually be false positives). The average life expectancy of a newly HIV-infected person is about 10 years.[7] This means that five or more years of premium income will be derived from the average newly enrolled infected person. If 1,000 tests produce two cases, and those two persons paid five years of premiums each (aggregating about $20,000), we can see that the cost of tests could well be more than the AIDS case costs less the premium revenues. Only if the testing produced a significantly higher yield of positive results than expected would the balance tip. That seemingly could happen only if the tests were required selectively— for example, by occupational category. In the United States, that would probably be found to be illegal. A number of states have enacted laws that either prohibit testing of health insurance applicants altogether, or prohibit discriminatory testing.[8]

Second, there is a terrible dilemma facing the insurer who, having required an applicant for coverage to submit to an HIV-antibody test, receives the report of a positive finding. There is surely a moral and almost certainly a legal obligation in this country to let the applicant know about that result. This is important not only for the applicant's sake but also to help assure that the applicant will not spread the infection to others. It is well understood, however, that it is highly inappropriate simply to put devastating information of this kind into an envelope to be mailed to the unsuspecting individual. Moreover, a single positive HIV-antibody test is not definitive proof of HIV infection. A repeat test is necessary, and, if it is also positive, a confirmative test is needed. Having learned about the first positive finding, the insurance plan has a patent moral duty at least to call the applicant back in for more tests to clarify whether that finding was genuine. Does the plan also have an obligation to report the positive finding to the public health authority? Should the applicant be given counseling? Should the applicant's spouse or other sex partners be notified? Should the applicant's personal physician be notified, and, if so, is the insurance plan under an obligation to pay for a physician visit? Questions such as these have helped persuade most insurers not to require testing of applicants.

2. *What services should health insurance cover for persons with AIDS?* In the United States, people covered

by health insurance have a large variety of specific different benefit plans, with a wide range of inclusions, exclusions, and limits. This question—What should the plans pay for?—is therefore really a question about whether insurance plans should consider excluding some benefits only for subscribers who have AIDS or whether to put in any special enlarged benefits just for such subscribers.

This question prompts another simple question—Why? What is there in AIDS that differs from other diseases that would warrant either special exclusions or special benefits? As we have seen, AIDS cases currently represent a minuscule fraction of the nation's health care burden; and AIDS-related care, spread over the average life expectancy of the newly HIV-infected individual, is not more costly than care for a fair number of other much more prevalent diseases.

Persons with AIDS typically do require periodic hospitalizations to deal with acute episodes of illness. The large bulk of the care that such people need, however, is more efficiently and humanely rendered in ambulatory, home, or hospice settings. This paper cannot deal with the evolution in treatment patterns that is taking place in the United States. That evolution, in any event, is one that emphasizes case management, reliance on voluntary community service infrastructures, and non-institutional services, including broader and earlier uses of some promising drugs. And it is resulting in lower per-year and lifetime costs.

Health insurance, on the other hand, traditionally tilts toward covering the costliest forms of care: hospitalization and the services of surgeons and other physicians who provide secondary and tertiary care. This suggests that many typical benefit plans may be less than adequate in dealing with AIDS patients' main needs for home and ambulatory care and prescription drugs. That's no doubt true, but not solely with respect to AIDS. There are many other chronic and degenerative diseases in which expensive acute care services are not the main need. The deficiencies in many benefit plans in providing meaningful protection for such persons are well-known.

Should insurance plans consider creating special benefits just for subscribers with AIDS, to cover medically appropriate home and ambulatory care and to underwrite the costs of professional case management? Such special benefits could well help to avert unneeded and costly hospitalizations, and thus could happily provide advantages for both the patients and the payers.

Yet, the number of persons with other diseases and disabilities that are best served in settings other than the hospital vastly exceeds the number of such persons with AIDS. Health economist and social critic Uwe Reinhardt has suggested that AIDS may be the catalyst to support changes in American health care delivery and insurance which will have impact far greater than on AIDS alone. If, in fact, an insurance plan's benefit patterns do a poor job in covering services needed by AIDS patients (who are few in number), they are doing an equally poor job with respect to more prevalent diseases that present similar medical care challenges to many more patients.

3. *Should insurance plans pay for experimental drugs and treatments for enrollees with AIDS?* Because HIV infection appears inexorably to lead to AIDS, and because AIDS appears inexorably to lead to death, it is highly understandable that many HIV-infected persons, even before they become ill, feel desperate. That desperation has led to an extensive underground network, both voluntary and entrepreneurial, to purchase and distribute unapproved and often untested drugs and food supplements.

Those materials would ordinarily not be covered by private health insurance plans in the United States because of clauses in their contracts excluding benefits for drugs and other treatments that are experimental and not approved by the appropriate federal authorities. That exclusion applies to drugs under development that are not yet cleared by the Food and Drug Administration for use and also to materials that are presented as being therapeutic but are not even under scientific evaluation.

For insurers, then, the issue seems straightforward. There seem to be no compelling reasons to make exceptions for AIDS patients for unapproved or experimental drugs, any more than there were when some cancer doctors in the 60s were demanding benefits for krebiozin and in the 70s were clamoring for laetrile. Exceptions for non-approved therapies constitute a slippery slope. How can a plan then avoid paying for unapproved therapies for a whole range of intractable diseases? How could AIDS defensibly be singled out?

4. *Should health insurance plans provide benefits for HIV-antibody tests?* The HIV-antibody test is medically vital for the individual who appears to have been exposed to the virus in a manner which could result in becoming HIV-infected. Most benefit plans, if they cover diagnostic laboratory studies at all, would automatically also cover the HIV-antibody test when ordered by a physician on the basis of a patient's likelihood of having been exposed, just as they would for other infectious diseases such as hepatitis or meningitis.

The more problematic issue arises from the fact that insurance plans in the United States ordinarily do not provide benefits for services that are rendered for public health purposes. If any employer or a unit of government, for example, wishes to have blocs of persons tested in order to identify infected individuals, most plans would not be obliged to provide benefits. Similarly, if surgeons or hospitals wish to test all patients in order to protect themselves from unknowing exposure to HIV, health insurance would not directly bear those costs.

As always, there are questions about borderlines. For example, authorities have urged HIV testing for certain population groups that may be at high risk, such as persons who received blood transfusions between 1978 and 1982. Here the answers are difficult to generalize across health insurance contracts' wide range of covered benefits for preventive services, including screening for relatively high-risk diseases. Again, at any rate, it is difficult to find a convincing rationale for paying for HIV screening while not paying for, say, mammograms for women as they get older.

5. *How can a plan protect itself against adverse selection when offering health insurance to persons not now covered?* The large majority of employed Americans are already covered by health insurance plans of one kind or another. This question therefore addresses a small minority within a minority: the person applying for benefits for the first time, whether as a new employee in a group for which the plan bears insurance risks or as a non-group direct-pay enrollee. If one insurer receives a disproportionate number of such persons who are HIV-infected, the consequence could be adverse claims experience that would drive premium rates above those of competing plans that avoided such enrollees. At the plan that employs me, we have indeed found that experience in the small-group market segment.

Traditionally, "pre-existing condition" clauses in their contracts are an insurer's main protection. Such clauses can be worded and interpreted in many different ways, but their effect is always to relieve the insurer of responsibility for the expenses of treatment of medical conditions that the subscriber had during a period prior to joining the plan. That relief is sometimes permanent, but more frequent in the non-profit plans are time-specific exclusions, such as 10- or 12-month periods after initial enrollment during which services related to the pre-existing condition are not covered.

Persons with AIDS therefore may be dissuaded from applying for enrollment in a health insurance plan by the knowledge that benefits will not be available for many months, precisely for the services that they will need.

As to HIV-infected persons who do not have AIDS at the time of enrollment, obtaining the results of AIDS antibody tests would provide a mechanism to identify such people in order to deny them enrollment in the plan. As discussed earlier, however, it is enormously costly to screen a random population for HIV infection using existing technology. It is for these sound business reasons that in 1988 the national Blue Cross and Blue Shield Association approved a report that pointed out to member plans the high costs and low results of using HIV-antibody testing to try to screen out infected applicants for insurance.[4] This position is in the process of being re-evaluated, however, because of the increasing treatment of HIV infection, in the absence of any other signs and symptoms, as an illness the course of which can frequently be altered by administering AZT or other costly medications.

In an arena as fiercely price-competitive as the small-group health insurance marketplace, carriers are pressured to keep premiums low through devices such as "medical underwriting" to identify high-risk people in advance. In fact, HIV infection is only one of hundreds of conditions that represent high risk and is numerically much rarer than many of the others. For insurers that do strict medical underwriting, there would seem to be little justification to exempt people with HIV infection from consideration for insurance.

NOTES

1. *Cancer Facts and Figures*, American Cancer Society, Atlanta, Georgia, 1989.

2. *AIDS Weekly Surveillance Report*, U.S. Public Health Service, Centers for Disease Control, Atlanta, Georgia. August 8, 1988.

3. Scitovsky AA and Rice DP. "Estimates of the Direct and Indirect Costs of Acquired Immunodeficiency Syndrome in the U.S., 1985, 1986, and 1991." *Public Health Reports* 102(1):5-17, January-February 1987 (data extrapolated by author).

4. *AIDS: A Resource Document for Blue Cross and Blue Shield Plans*. Blue Cross and Blue Shield Association, Chicago, Illinois, 1988.

5. Hellinger FJ. "Forecasting the Personal Medical Care Costs of AIDS from 1988 through 1991." *Public Health Reports* 103(3):309-319, May-June 1988.

6. Schramm CJ. "Insurers Advocate HIV Testing." *AIDS Patient Care* 2(1):4-6, February 1988.

7. Cowell MJ and Hoskins WH. *AIDS, HIV Mortality and Life Insurance*, Society of Actuaries, Schaumburg, Illinois, 1987.

8. Danler J. "Insurance Testing for HIV." *AIDS Patient Care* 2(1):11-13, February 1988.

QUESTIONS AND ANSWERS

The panelists answering questions included, in order of their workshop presentations:

Donald Young, MD, Executive Director, Prospective Payment Assessment Commission

Carl Schramm, PhD, JD, President, Health Insurance Association of America

Steven Sieverts, Vice President for Health Care Finance, Blue Cross and Blue Shield, National Capital Area

Additional comments by:

Charles Lewis, MD, ScD, Professor of Medicine, Public Health, and Nursing, School of Medicine, the University of California at Los Angeles

Q: (to panel) In Canada, insurance costs are as high as they are here, but the system is less acute care driven, far more equitable and comprehensive. Not only long-term care, but also more home care is covered. Here we have no system to handle paying for such additional costs as housing. Should we be modeling ourselves more after the Canadian approach?

A: (by Sieverts) At Blue Cross we do pay for more than short-term acute care medical costs. Prescription drugs, ongoing physician services, home care, and hospice care are all covered for chronic and long-term care, as well as acute care, for AIDS and other conditions. Nursing home care is about all that is not covered.

Comment: (by Schramm) In contrast to the level of hysteria about AIDS that we saw in the early to mid-1980s, now it's treated simply as "another disease" by insurance companies. There is no disparity between the policy for AIDS and the policy for other diseases, and it's hard to make the case that AIDS services should be specifically covered. The problem of insuring for AIDS is really just one aspect of a much larger health care financing problem, and it must be integrated into the big picture.

Q: (to panel) For AIDS, definitions about levels of care are problematic. Should it be treated as analogous to cancer?

A: (by Young) We shouldn't hide behind differences in diseases. We can't continue to say "Housing and hospice care are not my problem." The challenge is to cover hospice care, as Medicare now does.

Comment: (not identified) Medicaid spends four percent, or about $40 million of its budget on AIDS care. In Dallas, Texas, less than a third of the PWAs have no private insurance coverage.

Comment: (by Lewis) As a doctor, I'm very aware that physicians don't see the bills for materials we order for the patients we see, so we really are not able to participate in strategies for savings.

Q: (to panel) Are people with AIDS now living long enough to use up their financial resources so that their dying process isn't covered by insurance?

A: (not identified) This question is not specific to AIDS, but a more general problem.

Q: (to panel) What is happening with the pre-existing condition issue? How would this affect payments for AZT?

A: (by Sieverts) There is an issue as to whether HIV infection, short of any symptoms, should be considered an "illness." If it is not, then medications used "prophylactically" would generally be excluded from benefits. If HIV infection were defined as an illness, then we would pay for early administration of AZT, but would consider HIV infection to be a pre-existing condition with respect to new enrollees.

There is some abuse with respect to pre-existing condition clauses. The way they are set up now, some employers change health insurance carriers every year, so that employees face new pre-existing condition requirements, thus lowering the employer's costs. One finds some aggressive brochures and agents who encourage this practice, which is actually illegal in New York and perhaps in other states, too.

EDUCATION, TREATMENT, AND PAYMENT PRESSURES ON THE FEDERAL AND STATE GOVERNMENTS: PRESENTATIONS AND PANEL DISCUSSION

Structural Barriers to Financing Early Intervention and Treatment for AIDS
Timothy Westmoreland

Problems in Administering the HRSA AIDS Programs: Short-term, Unpredictable and Rigid Funding Constraints
Judith B. Braslow

The Community Health Center Program
Richard C. Bohrer

Failures in Public Policy and the Crisis in HIV Care and Treatment in the United States, 1990
Robert F. Hummel

AIDS and the Medicaid Program: A View from the States
Gary J. Clarke

The Role of the States in Providing Financing and Access to HIV and AIDS Health Care Services
Richard E. Merritt

□ Questions and Answers

Closing Statement
Paul S. Jellinek, PhD

STRUCTURAL BARRIERS TO FINANCING
EARLY INTERVENTION AND TREATMENT FOR AIDS

Timothy Westmoreland

My purpose today is to sort out the roles and responsibilities of the federal government in regard to AIDS. It's clear that problems of health care finance for AIDS at the federal level are both structural and fiscal. Money is a major issue, but the lack of coordinated planning among public health, biomedical research, and finance agencies is also a major problem that has been crystallized by the AIDS epidemic. Health care financing agencies pay for acute care but do not budget for prevention and public health—either for AIDS or for the other public health problems. Public health problems often intersect with health care financing issues with ferocity. In the past, tuberculosis, teen pregnancy, and lead screening programs have been served very badly by health care financing. However, AIDS has thrown the financing problem into bold relief with particular immediacy and an unforgiving clarity and insistence.

Structural Barriers to Health Care Financing

A quick response to AIDS care has been hampered by the fact that federal financing decision makers are used to working with data systems and data sets that are three to five years old. The momentum of AIDS puts such information out of date very rapidly; bulletins from the epidemic come in by the month. Strategic planning is further hindered by the fact that we are planning for delivery of drugs whose cost and effectiveness are not fully understood. Indeed, in many ways, we must plan for delivery of therapies that haven't even been discovered yet. But the force of the epidemic is so great that if financing systems aren't in place when these therapies become available, it will be too late.

The federal structure is poorly equipped for such intersections of public health and financing. In the early years of AIDS, the Centers for Disease Control (CDC) saw itself as a medical SWAT team, doing short-term, directed work. By contrast, the National Institutes of Health (NIH) thought of itself as a medical university—doing long-term, non-directed work, arriving at answers by Brownian motion and freedom of inquiry.

With the arrival of AIDS, there was a major gap, because neither agency considered the necessary long-term, directed epidemic research as its responsibility. It has taken a long time for CDC and NIH to recognize that the expertise of both agencies is needed for this kind of research. Now, of course, they have met in the middle, and CDC is doing long-term public health work while NIH is performing directed research.

A similar lack of policy intersection now exists between the Health Care Financing Administration (HCFA) and the Public Health Service (PHS). The PHS has done its job in identifying the epidemic, projecting its scope, identifying risk groups, and beginning to find treatments. Yet the PHS has not found a way to make these treatments available to the poor and uninsured.

The PHS has been unable to do so, because the Office of Management and Budget, the White House, and the Secretary of Health and Human Services have assigned responsibility for health care access to

Since 1979, Timothy Westmoreland has served as counsel to the Subcommittee on Health and the Environment of the Energy and Commerce Committee, United States House of Representatives.

HCFA. Yet HCFA has been getting no real direction or leadership on how to provide AIDS health care and therefore has been in a holding pattern—writing policy proposals that assume no real change in beneficiaries, services, or even costs.

The lack of communication and coordination between the PHS and HCFA has led to a situation where the advances that have been made in our ability to predict the epidemic and provide treatment have not been translated into services to people. So, for example, while we know that early intervention with AZT is useful, it is unavailable to the poor. As a result, there is a growing financing crisis and health care gridlock seen in the following ways, among others:

☐ AIDS incidence and mortality rates soar among the uninsured, even as they slow among the insured, according to recent NIH studies.

☐ Public hospitals overflow with acutely ill patients.

☐ Emergency rooms are forced to deal with AIDS primary care.

☐ While clinics and consortia demonstrate excellent AIDS care models, no long-term financing is available to them.

Finding a Way Out

It's difficult to envision the way out of this situation. Recent federal budgets don't take into account the growing AIDS health care costs which are much more expensive than educational pamphlets or even research projects. In some quarters, opinion is nearing a backlash—a perception that favoritism has been shown to AIDS patients. There is little understanding of the structural problems in public health care delivery generally, which AIDS merely highlights.

This situation is exacerbated by the changing epidemiology of AIDS as it moves into disenfranchised groups. Therefore, it's likely that there will be a political tendency for federal financing agencies to let HIV and AIDS smoulder as a public health problem, as has been done with tuberculosis, hypertension, teen pregnancy, and lead poisoning.

Viewed solely from a political angle, one change that may produce action has been that the distribution of AIDS has become more geographically widespread. It is no longer perceived as limited to far-away urban areas.

Early Intervention—A Top Priority

As we attempt to solve the structural dilemma of a lack of intersection between health care finance and public health, our first approach must be to keep things from getting even worse than they are right now. With this in mind, health care financing should take a dose of preventive medicine—with the public health approach that an ounce of early intervention is worth a pound of hospital care.

Right now, people are relieved at the possibility that—according to recent CDC estimates—"only" one million people may be HIV-infected. But consider the fact that the CDC, NIH, and the Defense Department are projecting that 51 percent of those now HIV-infected have T-cells below 500—reflecting the fact that their immune systems are dangerously weak. These people are very likely to get ill soon.

We need to find a way to make sure that when these HIV-infected people do develop symptoms, they get the early intervention drugs we've spent the last year and a half developing. They can't wait until we have national health insurance. Medicaid doesn't provide for early intervention because it requires that people be fully disabled before they are eligible for coverage. However, through early intervention, health care providers hope to delay full disability for those with AIDS. HCFA must do more to encourage early intervention treatment—aerosol pentamidine and AZT and, we hope, Fluconazol—soon enough to be useful to patients. At the same time, in a sort of mutual feedback, NIH must do more research into early interventions that will reduce the need to hospitalize people with AIDS.

The importance of early intervention is underlined by the hospitals' current struggle to pay for 50,000 living AIDS patients. By 1991, they will face 100,000. The only way these hospitals can survive is if not all the one million HIV-infected people get sick.

Representative Henry Waxman (D-CA), chair of the House Energy and Commerce Committee's Health Subcommittee for which I work, will be proposing legislation this year which we hope will begin to address these problems. It will provide grants to do counseling and testing, diagnostics, and early intervention through community-based clinics.

The bill also calls for changes in Medicaid that will give states the ability to make immuno-compromised, very poor people eligible for benefits before they're fully disabled. This would not be a change in poverty standards, but it would begin to provide some access to early intervention while it's still useful to people.

In supporting early intervention, it is important to remember one unfortunate approach to financing that exists—the "cheaper to let them die" mentality. It is illustrated by an early 1980s HCFA memo regarding the costs of covering pneumococcal pneumonia vaccine. The concern was not that paying for the vaccine under Medicare would be expensive, because people might have adverse reactions to it. Instead, the concern was that expense would arise, because the elderly people who got it would live longer and therefore continue to collect more health benefits. That mentality has a strong undertow, as we discuss the relationship between health care financing and public health.

Emergency Assistance—Acute Care for AIDS

However, early intervention alone won't stop the growing HIV and AIDS caseload—first, because the drugs aren't that good; second, because many people will still not receive them; and third, because many people are already too sick to benefit. Therefore, the federal government also needs to do much more to support direct, acute care for AIDS patients.

One approach would be to provide immediate emergency assistance. On Capitol Hill, emergency aid assistance is being discussed for high AIDS-incidence cities: If it's good enough for earthquakes, it should be good enough for viruses. Although not a long-term solution, emergency assistance would provide an immediate infusion of cash for areas having cash-flow problems in helping people with AIDS.

A cautious approach must be taken with emergency aid in order to avoid simply supplanting state and local efforts with federal dollars. You don't want just to buy the same services with a different checking account. It's also important to be sure that acute and long-term care demands don't become so pressing that money for prevention and community services is crowded out.

Past experience also indicates that no-strings, quick-access money can poison the well for future services—that if these funds are given out with no planning, no reporting, and no questions asked, there will be problems. Misuses, abuses, or losses—even small ones—can drive other future funders away.

In addition to emergency funds for acute AIDS care, many actions need to be taken affecting Medicaid and private payors. For hospitals that serve a disproportionate share of AIDS patients, disproportionate

Medicaid monies need to be made available. All hospitals lose money on Medicaid patients. Hospitals with AIDS Medicaid patients lose alot of money.

We must also stop the shift of financial responsibility from private sector insurance companies to public sector hospitals and payment systems. The easiest and most direct approach would be to allow Medicaid to pay premiums for continuation insurance required by the Consolidated Omnibus Budget Reconciliation Act (COBRA). We also need to make available home and community-based AIDS services for children through Medicaid without requiring that such programs demonstrate budget neutrality.

All these are complex issues that require debate. The real overall issue, however, is that financing agencies have not heard the public health message. Although we know the epidemic's impact is coming, we aren't preparing for it very well. The best way we can reverse that is with an ounce of prevention.

Problems in Administering the HRSA AIDS Programs: Short-term, Unpredictable and Rigid Funding Constraints

Judith B. Braslow

The lack of coordination between public health service programs and the federal health care financing system was described vividly in Tim Westmoreland's presentation. The day-to-day results of this structural problem are manifest in many ways as we attempt to develop and administer mandated AIDS and other public health programs through the Health Resources and Services Administration (HRSA). Funding may be too short-term to bring satisfactory outcomes, too unpredictable to allow for future planning, or too rigid to take into account expanding needs. Current government priorities naturally play a part in how to allocate scarce funding as well.

For example, The AIDS Pediatric Demonstration Program, which is administered by the Office of Maternal and Child Health, receives proportionately more money than the Office of Special Projects-administered AIDS Service Demonstration Projects, which focus on adults. When I'm asked why this is so, I can only say that the HIV problem in mothers and children is being given a high federal priority at this time, as reflected in actions of the congressional appropriations committees. This is a legislative decision as opposed to one made by the Public Health Service (PHS).

Problems with Start-stop Funding

Short-term funding and lack of predictable funding make planning, administration, and program assessment difficult and create frustration among grantees. HRSA AIDS Programs for which start-stop funding is a problem and which will probably be one-year efforts include: the HIV Services Planning Program, the Home Health Services Program, the Subacute Care Demonstration Program, and the Drug Reimbursement Program.

The HIV Services Planning Program—which provides year-long planning grants for 12 cities and 10 states—has only one year of funding. In addition, funding that had been allocated by both houses of Congress for additional planning grants in FY 1990 was eliminated in conference. When I go to meetings with our planning grantees, they ask if monies will be available to implement their planning documents, and I have no answer for them.

Because the congressional authorization for the Home Health Services Program and the Subacute Care Demonstration Program both expire at year-end, no new monies have been allocated in the President's budget. Therefore, at HRSA we are now in the position of announcing availability of funds and getting the programs off the ground, while at the same time having no authorization or budgeted funds for programs in their second year. We don't know what will happen, but right now our best guess is that these will be one-year-only programs.

Judith B. Braslow is acting director, Office of Special Projects, Bureau of Maternal and Child Health and Resources Development, Health Resources and Services Administration, U.S. Department of Health and Human Services.

Start-stop funding also continues to be a problem for the Drug Reimbursement Program. That program has received 11th hour funding every year for three years now, so planning and assessment have been very difficult.

Programs with Longer-term Funding, but Rigid Constraints

The Services Demonstration Program and the Education and Training Centers Program are the only two programs in the AIDS arena that have had some continuity of support. With fairly level funding since 1986, we are able to predict that the Services Demonstration Program will continue to be supported as an on-going program. The 1990 budget is $17.2 million, with $16.3 million actually available to appropriate to grantees. (Administration and one percent sequestered evaluation funds take the rest.)

While stable funding sounds like good news, for this program the financial pressures are tremendous. We have approximately the same level of funding that we had in 1986 with *four* grantees. Yet now we have 25 grantees. For nine of the grantee sites, The Robert Wood Johnson Foundation has spent an additional total of $17.1 million in funding, but that comes to an end this year. When we examine our total funding for this year, we actually have about $29 million out in the field. Next year we will have only the $16.3 million, yet we will have additional programs to which we've committed funding.

In order to meet our commitment of some funding to all 25 current programs, we will have to do some serious priority-setting. Probably we'll have to say we can only fund core services and eliminate necessary but lower priority services, such as transportation or meals-on-wheels.

The Facilities Renovation Program, also known as the 16.10(b) Program, has some stable funding. However, it suffers from structural rigidity of another kind. The most crucial facilities need is to house AIDS patients. Yet this program, funded under the Hill-Burton authority, requires that medical services be offered at any facility to be funded. Many applications come in that are clearly trying to provide group homes or congregate housing, but they are forced to demonstrate that they are also going to offer medical services. It's too early to evaluate the program, because the renovations have taken time to complete. However, it's safe to say that the Facilities Renovation Program does not address the housing needs of AIDS patients as efficiently as it could.

The final AIDS-related HRSA program is the Community Health Center Program, which is recently funded. Its purpose will be to fund AIDS services through community and migrant health centers. Since this program is new, it is too early to tell whether it will receive stable funding or whether it will be able to provide services successfully. (Note: This program is discussed further in the next paper by Richard Bohrer.)

THE COMMUNITY HEALTH CENTER PROGRAM

Richard C. Bohrer

The Health Care Services Program

Judith Braslow has just discussed the budgetary situation of the HRSA AIDS programs. I would like to elaborate a bit on the last program she mentioned, the Community Health Center Program.

Since 1988, our health centers have experienced roughly a 60 percent increase in the number of HIV-infected and AIDS patients served. In some states, these centers are a significant provider of care. For example, in states with relatively high caseloads, like Pennsylvania and Maryland, community and migrant health centers serve more than 10 percent of the identified AIDS patients.

The Community Health Center Program has funding for 1990 ($10.8 million) and also has requested money for 1991 ($13.3 million). Through this program, community and migrant health centers will be able to provide acute health services for HIV-infected and AIDS patients. In addition, they will offer counseling, case management, and prevention services.

The health centers targeted will be those in 30 or 40 communities where, based on CDC data, a significant incidence of HIV infection has already been seen. In addition, support will be given to health centers which are already actively involved in primary care activities for HIV and AIDS patients. We anticipate that the health centers will be part of networks of local public and private care and service providers, as well.

Problems in AIDS Care and Services—Structure and Finance

I would also like to reinforce what the past two speakers have said. That is, I wholeheartedly concur that the difficulties in confronting the issues of AIDS prevention and services are definite systemic problems of access. At the community delivery level, decisions must be made about how to spread limited resources as far as they will go; ultimately this translates into decisions about how best to serve people with equal health needs—for example, an HIV-infected person, a pregnant teen, someone with a drug problem, or an AIDS patient with the usual acute and chronic care needs.

Based on my 20 years with the Public Health Service, most of the time it's difficult to get people to recognize that in order to address a public health problem, more than financing is involved. Whether the need is for primary, secondary, or tertiary health services, solutions must be not only through finance, but also through structure and capacity-building.

Assistant Surgeon General Richard C. Bohrer is the director of the Division of Primary Care Services, Bureau of Health Care Delivery and Assistance, in the Health Resources and Services Administration (HRSA), U.S. Department of Health and Human Services.

FAILURES IN PUBLIC POLICY AND THE CRISIS IN HIV CARE AND TREATMENT IN THE UNITED STATES, 1990

Robert Hummel

Introduction

In 1983, I was one of three people at the New York State Department of Health AIDS Institute—it now has a staff of over 250 and a budget of $60 million. From my perspective, as someone who has been around since the beginning, we're moving towards the tenth anniversary of this epidemic in the midst of complete moral bankruptcy in public policy and public health strategy. We are, in fact, in a public policy vacuum in this country.

I see the problem as analogous to the situation during the Vietnam War, when the United States government failed to have an agreed-upon strategy. Part of the reason is that we conveniently call this an "AIDS epidemic," which keeps the numbers down, when actually we are in the midst of an HIV epidemic. In New Jersey, no one gets too upset about 7,000 or 8,000 diagnosed AIDS cases, but they would take notice of 50,000 to 70,000 HIV-infected individuals.

As with the Vietnam War, we're saying, "Okay, we won; let's go home." We are beginning to mainstream HIV and AIDS, to compare them to other diseases, and to say, "Oh, it's not so bad after all." In the meantime, it's still an epidemic, and if we don't act, we'll pay for it in the future. Cancer and heart disease will not increase in the same manner as will HIV and AIDS unless we intervene with strong public policy and strong prevention and service programs.

Failures in HIV Public Policy

American public policy has failed in a number of areas. First, after 10 years, we still don't have an accurate idea of how many people are being infected with HIV daily. Therefore, we have no way of making a rational response or developing a strategy that we can expect will be appropriate even into the next year.

Second, for years and years we've been talking about the need for financial restructuring, for housing, and for collateral services, and we still have not taken adequate action. In the meantime, thousands—hundreds of thousands—of people have been infected and need services. The big metropolitan areas have been a bellwether for what the whole nation will face in the future, and the biggest increases will be in areas that haven't yet been hit with HIV.

Third, we are dealing with a bureaucratic maze. The leadership vacuum for HIV and AIDS policy has left us with budget analysts who have no public-policy training to make program and policy decisions. I actually had one financial analyst say to me, in regard to the New Jersey Treatment Assessment Program, "Well, it would be cheaper to let them die, wouldn't it?" Values like these—rather than fairness, justice and humanity—are being brought into play in making AIDS policy.

Since 1988, Robert Hummel has served as assistant commissioner for AIDS Prevention and Control, New Jersey Department of Health.

Finally—and frankly I'm surprised that this issue hasn't been discussed more at this meeting—is the decimation of minority and disenfranchised populations by HIV and AIDS. The epidemic is now becoming less associated with risk groups and more related to socioeconomic factors.

The numbers game, as with the Vietnam War, allows you to pick whatever numbers you want to make your point, but regardless of whether the number is 50,000 or 100,000 HIV-infected drug addicts in Newark, we are unprepared, and we are facing a major public policy and programmatic catastrophe.

The Crisis in Care and Treatment

Along with the public policy vacuum, we also face a crisis in HIV and AIDS care and treatment. The states, and especially the high incidence states, cannot absorb the cost of care and treatment for this epidemic. Therefore, it was unconscionable for CDC to announce last summer the effectiveness of aerosol pentamidine and AZT for early intervention and at the same time say that such care must be state-financed.

The difficulty in AIDS financing is clearly demonstrated in the state of New Jersey. There, we have an uncompensated care fund of $500 million for all residents who are uninsured or underinsured. Yet the 1992 cost for diagnosed AIDS cases alone is expected to be $1 billion—twice the money in the uncompensated care fund.

The federal government must recognize that we can no longer talk about HIV prevention without also talking about access to early intervention. Clinical research has led us to the point where it is imperative that policymakers and public health officials take responsibility for developing such care programs. I want to emphasize that, for these programs, grants and start-stop funding are totally inappropriate. With care and treatment, you can't put people on a roller coaster. There must be steady reimbursement streams.

The New Jersey Treatment Assessment Program

Despite public policy failures, and despite the care and treatment crisis, it's also true that in this country we do have HIV and AIDS-related programs that work, for example at Johns Hopkins in Baltimore. In New Jersey, a program I am involved in developing is also proving successful in its early stages. It is the Treatment Assessment Program (TAP), started in October 1989 at the Jersey City Medical Center with $200,000. As of now, the TAP program is state-wide, with five sites around the state.

At the Jersey City Medical Center Program, a reported 435 clients—40 percent black, 30 percent Hispanic, and 30 percent white—participated during the first three months. They came mainly after hearing about it by word of mouth—proving that people in a drug-using population will come forward. While the data are much too preliminary for publication, suffice it to say that we have found the numbers shockingly high. More than half of the 435 proved symptomatic at some level, and, of these, many had T-cell counts below 500 and are now on AZT therapy. The large percent with T-cell counts below 200 are on *Pneumocystis carinii* pneumonia (PCP) prophylaxis, and most are on Bactrum and Septra. Fifteen percent are on aerosol pentamidine.

We are surprised at the high compliance rate and rate of return visits, since this is not typical of a drug-using population. For TAP clients, we also see lower hospital admissions and readmissions and reduced length of stay because of the effectiveness of outpatient management.

Although our financial projections are extremely tentative, we anticipate an average cost of $3,000 annually for a TAP client. If we can avoid one acute admission for PCP per client, that reduces inpatient costs by $10,000 for a non-drug user and $13,000 for a drug user.

We can't talk about "cost containment," because 435 people are in the system who weren't there previously, and they are going to cost money. But they may not cost more than they would have had they begun by presenting at the emergency room in acute episodes. What we can talk about is cost efficiency and appropriate utilization of services with fewer capital expenditures.

My big concern now is how we are going to continue to pay for the TAP program. My division's budget has been cut by $2 million in the last year and a half. With 435 people at one site in the first three months, I expect all five programs to reach their maximum enrollment by summer's end. Yet, compared to the need, the number we are serving is minuscule. These 435 people represent less than one percent of the 50,000 to 70,000 of the total universe of HIV-infected people who will need early intervention and long-term care services in New Jersey.

AIDS AND THE MEDICAID PROGRAM:
A VIEW FROM THE STATES

Gary J. Clarke

My mission is to discuss the HIV epidemic in the context of the Medicaid program which is now, and for the foreseeable future, the single largest payer of AIDS care. The report that I bring you contains both good news and bad news. The bad news you already know. While there is some evidence that the rate of growth in the epidemic is slowing down, the absolute number of persons affected by this disease is still growing at a very rapid rate—and so too are Medicaid costs. The good news is that at least from our perspective of looking at claims data, costs per patient are not (and never were) nearly as high as alleged in the literature and seem to be continuing to moderate.

First, the bad news. In the large urban states where most of the persons with HIV infection reside, there is no question that the disease has made a major impact on total Medicaid costs. In Florida, for instance, the state with the third largest number of AIDS cases, we estimate that HIV-related Medicaid costs have risen from virtually nothing in 1984 to about $37 million today. With HIV-related costs expected to roughly double each year for the next two years, that number is expected to be $147 million in 1992-93. Not unexpectedly, most of this growth is tied directly to the projected increases in AIDS cases in Florida.

The good news, however, is really quite good. In reviewing our paid-claims history, we found that the number of days of hospitalization for AIDS patients has averaged about 23 days per annum. That is considerably less than the 36 to 50 days (or more) alleged in much of the AIDS cost literature, which is used as the basis for making national cost estimates. We found the same phenomenon to be true with AZT. While the early literature estimated that the annual cost for effective treatment was $8,000, we spent only 21 percent of that amount (on average)—even when AZT was being distributed to only the sickest patients. The lower cost was due to less utilization and lower prices than anticipated.

Early returns on the cost-effectiveness of providing AZT for Medicaid patients in Florida are even more promising. In a recent study we conducted for our legislature, we found not only that drug costs were lower, but that hospital days were dramatically reduced as well. After payment for AZT began, hospital days for Medicaid patients with AIDS fell by 10.6 percent, with no appreciable increase in mortality. In total, including increased costs for paying for the drug, as well as additional hematologic and other testing, annual per capita Mediciad costs still fell slightly below both our historical and predicted costs for these patients (savings of about $725 per patient per year).

While further studies are needed and under way to document the long-term cost effects of AZT and other drug therapies, what the clinicians are telling us is on the horizon seems to be emerging very clearly from the claims data, as well. That is, AIDS (or more properly, HIV infection), is and will become much more of a chronic disease, requiring long-term management and resources.

When thought of as a chronic disease, two policy implications for the future of the Medicaid program as it relates to AIDS care seem clear. First, with the exception of certain cities, the number of AIDS patients compared to other Medicaid patients with chronic disease is really very small, and in comparative percentage terms seems likely to remain so. For instance, nationally, 73 percent of all Medicaid expenditures

Gary J. Clarke is the assistant secretary for Medicaid in the Florida Department of Health and Rehabilitative Services.

already are spent on persons with chronic diseases and impairments (the elderly, and the totally and permanently disabled). AIDS simply adds another disease to a long list, including cancer, stroke, heart disease, liver failure, Alzheimer's, trauma, and severe developmental disability. In a state that has the third highest number of AIDS cases, we believe the cost for AIDS care is currently about one percent of all expenditures, and probably will get no higher than four percent. For comparison purposes, fully six percent of our current budget is spent on about 3,100 persons who reside in institutional facilities for the mentally retarded.

A second important policy point emerges once we think of AIDS as a chronic disease. Traditional Medicaid programs, like all traditional health insurance programs, are not really geared toward cost-effective care for chronic illness. While Medicaid is certainly much better than Medicare when it comes to chronic conditions (drug coverage and long-term institutional care), I think it is fair to say that neither public nor private insurance does a really good job with chronic care. In part, the problem is our lack of creativity, and in part the problem is the very nature of insurance itself. That is, as insurers, each of us pays only when claims are submitted (and frequently tries to avoid payment with exclusions, limitations, prior approval and the like). In addition, few insurers have the leverage to encourage providers to change their overall behavior to accommodate the needs of persons with a particular chronic disease. Stated another way, we only pay how people practice, which in turn causes them to practice only how we pay!

What's necessary to break this Gordian knot with regard to the Medicaid program is a combination of innovation at the state level and loosening of the regulatory strings at the federal level. Florida is one of approximately 10 states that has a home and community-based Medicaid waiver program for AIDS patients. We know from our own experience, from experience with the various Robert Wood Johnson Foundation and HRSA projects, and from the early experience in San Francisco on which we began modeling all of these programs, that home and community-based care is the way to go. It's more dignified, it's more comforting, it's more acceptable—and by the way—it's more cost-effective.

Requiring states to jump through complicated statutory hoops to do what we all believe is the right thing simply seems the wrong approach. In Florida, it took almost two years to get our waiver approved (granted, it's the largest in the country). At the very least, waiver services for AIDS (and I suggest, other chronic diseases) should be able to be picked up by the states as optional programs. With states sharing in the cost of care, HCFA can rest assured that the management of these programs will be as prudent as any other in Medicaid.

Medicaid waiver programs alone, however, will not guarantee acceptable, cost-effective treatment of AIDS and HIV-infected patients. Additional investments need to be made in those institutions where providers do the bulk of the care. Our experience in Florida, and, I think, the experience in New Jersey and now some of the big cities, portends the wave of the future of this epidemic. In the future, the AIDS epidemic will be concentrated among the poor, minorities, and drug abusers—and, most tragically, their children.

So, too, care for patients with AIDS will be concentrated among those health care institutions and practitioners who provide most of the care to these groups—teaching and public hospitals, community health and mental health clinics, health departments, and a smattering of private practitioners. Yet these health care institutions are the very least able to raise or to risk capital to provide care in new ways. Medicaid payments alone are not sufficient to encourage them to do this—even if everyone were covered.

As a result, start-up capital and ongoing support are necessary for these traditional providers of care to minorities and the poor. While AIDS may be the rationale, in my opinion, the truth is simply that AIDS is the proverbial straw that is breaking the camel's back. Any other epidemic, or even an economic recession, would have had the same effect. Yet AIDS is the precipitous event, and the result is that some of our finest and most critical institutions for serving minorities and the poor are groaning under the weight of their collective burden. In fact, I believe they are in serious danger of breaking down altogether.

While special grant support and home and community-based Medicaid services are needed, so, too, are other improvements in the Medicaid program. While I believe the problem with Medicaid "under-payment" of hospitals has been greatly exaggerated, other critical problems must be addressed. These problems include inordinately low rates of physician payments, low rates of payment for other non-institutional services, such as home health services, and a number of arbitrary limitations and caps. Limitations on hospital days (of from 12 to 45 days annually) are particularly common in southern Medicaid programs, and are the most pervasive reason for hospital Medicaid losses due to AIDS in that region of the country.

Better payment rates by themselves, however, will not remove the stigma associated with Medicaid in the minds of many health care providers. Much work remains to be done to change provider attitudes—and Medicaid system performance—if we are going to build viable systems of care for AIDS patients. At the same time, we must understand that for the majority of AIDS patients (adult males), eligibility continues to be a function of federal government policies through the Social Security Income program. While it has been easy for many to castigate the states for reductions in the numbers of persons who are covered (a statistic that has reversed itself due to recent optional and mandated programs), states are not in charge of eligibility for this group. Rather, Medicaid programs mostly pay the health care bills for those made eligible by the Social Security Administration (with the exception of the "209(b)" states).

Despite the conventional wisdom restated by some at this conference that "It is all the states' fault that more AIDS patients are not eligible for Medicaid," if we hope to make more persons with AIDS eligible for Medicaid (and more obviously, Medicare), it is federal—not state—policies that must change. This is not only possible, but there is plenty of precedent for it. For example, kidney disease patients are comprehensively covered under Medicare. In the Medicaid program, pregnant women and children under six have much less restrictive eligibility standards than do all other recipients. For those who ask why do this for AIDS patients in lieu of patients with other types of disease, I ask, "Why not?" If AIDS care is truly a priority, then we have both the available mechanisms and the precedent to make the necessary public policy changes.

In conclusion, unless care for AIDS patients is comprehensively covered under the Medicare program, I think the following three trends are inevitable with regard to AIDS and the Medicaid program:

First, Medicaid coverage is likely to become an even larger payer of care for AIDS patients in the future. The disease is more and more concentrated among the poor. As with many other diseases, its spread is now primarily a result of the ignorance, hopelessness, and recklessness that poverty itself breeds (especially IV drug use). Until we can break this vicious cycle, the primary insurance program for the poor—Medicaid—will be the single largest payer for AIDS care. And its costs will grow as the disease grows.

Second, AIDS care will place increasing pressure on those institutions and health care providers that primarily serve the poor. It is here, rather than in the state or federal budgetary arenas, that AIDS will compete with pregnant women and children for attention. In many places in this country, there are simply not the facilities, the personnel, or the cash to do an adequate job on either priority. Increased Medicaid coverage or enhanced reimbursement for AIDS may ease the strain somewhat but will not alter the fundamental underlying problems of the inadequacy of our health care delivery system for poor Americans.

Third, and finally, the entire Medicaid program itself may be heading for a major federal/state showdown—particularly in the South—regardless of the AIDS crisis. AIDS itself is only a small blip on the screen of most state Medicaid programs. But the impact of recent federal mandates on the states, combined with health care inflation and the increasing unavailability of private health insurance, is difficult to underestimate. In our state alone, total Medicaid increases have averaged 27 percent per year for the past four years—compared to overall revenue growth of seven percent. Despite accounting for 10 percent of the state budget, the Medicaid program in Florida will require 40 percent of all new state revenues this year just to stay in place and comply with new federal mandates. (If proposed, but not yet enacted, tax increases are not counted, 63 percent of all new revenue must be devoted to the Medicaid program to avoid cutbacks in eligibility or services.)

While we have made rapid strides to build an adequate Medicaid program in our state and in many places throughout the country, I believe the twin fuels of expanded eligibility and other mandates, plus health care inflation, are cooking a mixture few state legislatures have the ability to control. I worry that at some time in the not-too-distant future, a state will simply tell the federal government, "Here, you can have this program back. I can't afford it anymore, no matter how much good it does." If that happens, AIDS care will certainly not be the cause. Rather, it will be much larger health care economic problems that are at work, of which AIDS is only a small, though significant, part. Should such a turn-back of responsibility occur, I, for one, worry about the ability of the federal budget to come up with the billions of dollars states currently contribute to the program. More important, I worry about the care our recipients will receive.

THE ROLE OF THE STATES IN PROVIDING FINANCING AND ACCESS TO HIV AND AIDS HEALTH CARE SERVICES

Richard E. Merritt

AIDS Policy—Consensus within the States

As director of the Intergovernmental Health Policy Project, I have been able to develop an overview of the whirlwind of state legislative activity dealing with AIDS issues over the last seven or eight years. I'm pleased to say that, despite the controversial issues that generate much debate, overall, the AIDS crisis has not been highly politicized. At the state level, the amount of rancor has been kept to a minimum, and the amount of consensus has been rather amazing. In fact, I think it's fair to say that the preponderance of state enactments and policies have been reasonable, measured, and supportive of good public health goals.

By and large, states have rejected as false the idea that there is a dichotomy between personal liberties and the state's right to protect the public. While some states lean more in one direction or the other, most have worked to preserve a balance between individual and public rights.

For example, despite all the media attention to mandatory testing, to isolation, quarantine, contact tracing and the rest, few states have enacted laws in these areas. Rather than mandatory testing, the consensus is for voluntary testing based on written informed consent that includes pre-test and post-test counseling bolstered by strong protection of confidentiality.

Health Care Financing—A Three-legged Stool

As has been described several times today, we have a serious problem of fragmentation in the health care financing system. Let me describe what has been said in a slightly different way. Larry Brown at Harvard has described our health care financing system as a three-legged stool. The financing "legs" are:

☐ through fringe benefits in the workplace for most people

☐ through categorical entitlement for many others, and

☐ through chance and charity for the rest.

Unfortunately, each leg is fragmented within itself. Take private insurance: The Health Insurance Association of America represents about 300 different plans, while Blue Cross-Blue Shield has about 70 plans. We've already talked about the lack of uniformity in the Medicaid system, and the state safety net systems are even more complex and diverse than Medicaid. Charity care is fragmented among public hospitals, volunteer services, and various local agencies and groups.

In addition to fragmentation, the stability of each of the three "legs" of the financing stool is being whittled away. First, as the economy shifts from a manufacturing to a service base, employer-based insurance protections are eroding for many. Second, Medicaid serves less than 50 percent of those below the

Richard E. Merritt is the director of the Intergovernmental Health Policy Project at The George Washington University, where he is also on the faculty of the Department of Health Services Administration.

poverty index—a far lesser percentage than 10 years ago. And, finally, the informal safety net of providing uncompensated care through surcharges on private paying patients is under attack. Hospitals cannot continue to subsidize so much of the financing for poor people's care and remain financially viable.

People with HIV/AIDS—Victims of Financing Fragmentation and Erosion

People with HIV and AIDS are victims of this health care financing fragmentation and erosion and are very much at risk for becoming a subgroup of the overall growing population of indigent and uninsured. Their victimization is compounded by the nature of their disease—far too few providers are equipped and willing to care for these individuals.

Unfortunately, there's a consensus that has run through the federal health care financing system for years that, while entitlement can be tied to age or income, it should not be tied to a specific disease. The major exception was the program for end-stage renal disease begun in the early 1970s. Analysts agree that it was a cost-escalation disaster, and given the federal deficit, I think no further such disease-based entitlements are likely to be forthcoming.

On a more positive note, there is greater sensitivity and awareness nationally than ever before to the growing problems of the uninsured and indigent—of which those with HIV disease are a growing sub-population. The Pepper Commission and the Steelman Commission reflect this growing concern, in that both have been charged with recommending needed changes in the nation's health care system to expand access and control costs. In addition, polls show that Americans are in favor of a system more like the Canadian universal coverage system—although it's likely that the vast majority of those polled don't have a clear understanding of that system.

States Move towards Universal Coverage

Considerable activity has been taking place over the past few years at the state level to improve health care coverage for the uninsured. For example, Hawaii can lay claim to being the first state with almost universal access to health care for its entire population. Massachusetts has enacted the Health Security Act, which moves the state toward universal coverage over a several year phase-in period; Washington state is considering legislation modeled on the Canadian system; and Oregon has adopted a plan (which will require federal approval for it to be implemented) that calls for rationing certain health services while expanding Medicaid eligibility and private health insurance coverage. Half a dozen other states have proposals before their legislatures that would expand coverage for the indigent and uninsured.

In addition, Medicaid expansions over the past few years have focused on increasing coverage for pregnant women and children. More states are providing case management and home and community-based care under Medicaid—services which are particularly relevant to people with HIV and AIDS. Also, a few states have modified their reimbursement methods for hospital and nursing home services under Medicaid to increase access for AIDS patients.

Financing through Employers and through State Risk Pools

States are looking for better ways of maintaining and expanding employer-based health insurance for people with HIV disease as well. One approach is to assist individuals who are currently covered under a group policy to exercise their option granted under the Consolidated Omnibus Budget Reconciliation Act of 1985. Under this option, companies must allow recently terminated employees the ability to continue their health insurance coverage under the group policy for up to 18 months. The employee, however, is responsible for paying the full premium. Michigan, for example, is actually subsidizing the premiums of individuals with HIV disease who are likely to be disabled within three months. Eligibility is limited to those who have incomes below 200 percent of the poverty index and less than $10,000 in assets. Washington, Colorado, California, and a few other states are looking quite seriously at similar approaches.

In addition, states are encouraging small firms to offer health insurance. This is especially important, since individuals at greatest risk for HIV infection may be disproportionately represented among the self-employed and in small businesses. Incentives to small businesses that states may offer include providing tax incentives and authorizing less comprehensive benefit packages.

States are also focusing on the needs of the uninsurable population—that is, those with an existing condition that is likely to require extensive and expensive care in the future. Practically all insurance companies view HIV infection as an uninsurable condition.

One response is the creation of a state health insurance risk pool for otherwise uninsurable people, with all insurers doing business in the state (except the self-insured) required to cooperate in offering a comprehensive policy and to share in the financial losses. These policies are characterized by very high deductibles and co-payments and expensive premiums, so while a risk pool may help to address the problem of availability for many uninsurable individuals, it does very little for the problem of affordability. Currently, 18 states have mandated the establishment of risk-pool programs.

A major impediment to the growth of the risk-pool approach is that the federal ERISA law prohibits states from requiring self-insured plans to participate in the pool. Consequently, the financing base for these pools becomes rather constricted, limiting them mostly to commercial insurance companies and Blue Cross plans.

State Funding for AIDS/HIV

The states themselves have not been reluctant to put up funds for AIDS, contrary to Carl Schramm's remarks earlier. In fact, 1989 state appropriations through general funds—not federal or matched dollars—were in excess of $250 million for AIDS research, programs, surveillance, education, and services. Combined with state Medicaid dollars (about another $450 million), the 1989 state contribution to AIDS was about three-quarters of a billion dollars. For fiscal year 1990, estimates show that state money for AIDS and HIV will exceed $1 billion.

There is a trend away from state funding of areas that are really the responsibilities of other levels of government, such as AIDS research and surveillance. Instead, more and more state dollars are going into direct patient care for indigent AIDS patients and into supporting various social services that are not generally financed through third-party mechanisms. In about 10 states, the amount of state money going for AIDS-related programs is about equal to the amount of federal money, and in eight others, state dollars actually exceed federal dollars.

Indirect Approaches to Ensuring Access

In addition to these direct approaches to financing for AIDS/HIV, states influence access to care in a number of indirect ways—for example, through preventing employment discrimination on the basis of risk factors. Several states prohibit use of HIV tests as a precondition of employment unless absence of HIV is proved to be a bona fide occupational qualification. In addition, in most states, handicapped rights acts now prevent employers from terminating someone's employment solely on the basis of their HIV-infected status.

States are also becoming more aggressive in regulating the insurance industry. For example, some states now prohibit health insurance companies from providing more restrictive coverage for AIDS, ARC, or HIV infection than for other diseases. Many states forbid companies from canceling or failing to renew a health insurance policy because someone becomes diagnosed with AIDS while they are already covered by insurance.

Finally, states are working to curb discrimination against HIV-infected people by health care providers. After all, even with financing, access to care is not guaranteed. Probably the most stringent state law at the moment is in Maryland, where health care providers found guilty of refusing treatment to anyone with HIV disease can actually lose their licenses. Several other states have slightly less stringent regulations. In Rhode Island and Vermont, for example, health care providers cannot condition the provision of services on the basis of a patient's willingness to take an HIV test.

Conclusion

The state role in financing services for HIV and AIDS will grow in significance over the next few years as private insurers find more ways to limit their exposure, and as the populations affected shift towards intravenous drug users, urban minorities, and pediatric cases—groups which have traditionally been more reliant on public support. I believe that this growth in state financing will occur, however, not so much out of an attempt to meet the specific financial needs of those with HIV and AIDS, but rather as part of a more comprehensive approach to addressing the overall problems of the indigent and uninsured.

QUESTIONS AND ANSWERS

The panel for this question and answer period, in order of appearance below, was:

Richard Bohrer, Director, Division of Primary Care Services, Public Health Service, U.S. Department of Health and Human Services

Judith Braslow, Acting Director, Office of Special Projects, Bureau of Maternal and Child Health and Resources Development, DHHS

Timothy Westmoreland, Counsel, Subcommittee on Health and the Environment, Committee on Energy and the Environment, U.S. House of Representatives

Robert Hummel, Assistant Commissioner, Division of AIDS Prevention and Control, New Jersey State Department of Health

Gary Clarke, Assistant Secretary for Medicaid, State of Florida

Richard E. Merritt, Director, Intergovernmental Health Policy Project at The George Washington University

Additional comments were made by:

Cheryl Austein, Director, Division of Public Health Policy, Office of the Assistant Secretary for Planning and Evaluation, DHHS

Judith Miller Jones, Director, National Health Policy Forum, Washington, DC

Leighton Cluff, MD, President, The Robert Wood Johnson Foundation

Paul Jellinek, PhD, Senior Program Officer, The Robert Wood Johnson Foundation

Mervyn Silverman, MD, Director, AIDS Health Services Program, University of California at San Francisco

Ron Anderson, MD, Chief Executive Officer, Parkland Hospital, Dallas, TX

Patricia McInturff, Director, Regional Division, Seattle-King County Health Department

Donald Young, MD, Executive Director, Prospective Payment Assessment Commission

Steven Young, Director, Care and Treatment Unit, Division of AIDS Prevention and Control, New Jersey State Department of Health

Sister Rosemary Donley, RN, PhD, Executive Vice President, Catholic University of America, Washington, DC

Q: (to Bohrer by Jones) Let's assume for a moment that we do legislate an expansion of Medicaid for AIDS purposes. Would it be likely that we would tell the community health centers that they must collect these Medicaid payments and, therefore, that a reduction in their overall appropriation would be made?

A: (by Bohrer) That certainly would be discussed. As an example, this year there is a change in funding for "Federally Qualified Health Centers." This legislation allows health centers to be reimbursed by Medicaid for their costs for the first time. As we prepare budgets to support these centers, we must ask what the impact of that law will be. The question will be asked whether this potential $30 to $50 million dollars in Medicaid reimbursements that will be going to local health centers can be offset against their grants.

I think we can counter this idea because now the problems in access to health care are more visible, and, therefore, we clearly have a commitment within the Department of Health and Human Services to expand the community health centers' capacity.

Comment: (by Austein) Another example of how enhanced Medicaid reimbursement has impacted the Public Health Services is with infant mortality. A rapid expansion in Medicaid eligibility occurred at the same time we were putting additional public health money into community health centers and other programs serving disadvantaged pregnant women, mothers, and infants.

But now we must answer a difficult question: Are we truly expanding access and serving new patients through this increase in Medicaid, or are these the same patients who came in before, when they didn't have any health insurance? We tried to answer that question on a pilot basis, but the data are limited.

Comment: (by Jones) When one kind of dollar is substituted for another, it may not be of equal value. A Medicaid dollar is restricted to paying for only certain services. However, a dollar going directly to a community health center can provide many additional services that would never be reimbursed through Medicaid.

Comment: (by Braslow) As an example of how we in public health have worked with that, in the perinatal program we have allowed the Medicaid reforms to expand the core set of traditional services for pregnancy. Then, we have wrapped less traditional services—such as community outreach—around those provided by Medicaid using Community and Migrant Health Center monies. I'm optimistic that an argument for the same approach could be made for any population group for whom services and access are to be expanded.

Q: (by Cluff) It sounds as though many of the innovative programs I heard about yesterday are increasingly dependent on private, local, city, community, and state resources. I'm wondering how much coordination is going on between the federal and state levels.

A: (by Braslow) The only reason the HRSA Services Demonstration Program has been able to survive with level federal funding is because state and local funding has gone up. Because there is a lot of coordination, the money we have has been adequate to serve 25 sites—up from the four we originally had. In fact, I'd say the single greatest accomplishment of the HRSA Services Demonstration Program and our other AIDS programs has been the ability to leverage additional dollars.

For example, for the Facilities Renovation Program for AIDS, the 1988 figures were $6.7 million HRSA dollars leveraging $48 million state dollars. That's a pretty good investment of $6 million. However, although there's an enormous amount of coordination, I don't have to tell you the pressure the states are feeling.

Comment: (by Westmoreland) In the area of early intervention with prescription drugs, some states have been using state-only dollars to provide services. Although they're way out in front of federal policy, such states are few and far between. And for the "near poor," states have concentrated their efforts again on acute care and emergency situations rather than on early intervention.

Comment: (by Austein) Speaking as someone from an office within Health and Human Services (HHS) that does public health financing, I very much support what's been said. But I'd like to try to explain the dilemmas we face, given that our money is not unlimited.

☐ The Medicaid program has been asked to increase access to mothers and children.

☐ At the same time, the Medicare program is being asked to control expenditures for hospitals and doctors.

☐ Some groups are saying, increase access to drugs for HIV and AIDS patients—even though they may not be proven safe and effective. The Medicare program is supposed to cover drugs that are safe and effective and approved by FDA.

Comment: (by Westmoreland) I'd like to quickly respond to a couple of points. First, I'm not talking about the need for health care financing for experimental drugs, but for *approved* early-intervention drugs like aerosol pentamidine and AZT. Second, I understand that HCFA isn't responsible alone for the lack of funds. I know that Congress has been lax, too—in fact, many of the financing people in Congress don't talk to the financing people in the administration. This lack of coordination that goes on in academic discussions and at the state and local levels, definitely occurs with Congress as well.

Comment: (by Jellinek) Two quick points. First, the bottom-line issue with program and funding coordination is to get as much juice out of existing dollars as possible. It's important that we demonstrate that this is being done before allocating more money. Second, to the extent that we rely heavily on non-federal resources—state, local, and private dollars—communities will be at the mercy of local circumstances, which leads to questions of equity.

Q: (by Silverman to panel) I'd like the panel to discuss the fact that we don't have a clear idea of the nature, character, or magnitude of the HIV epidemic, except as measured by selected screening and testing procedures in the military, the blood banks, and with IV-drug abusers using treatment clinics like those in New Jersey. I know this is a key issue because of its enormous political, cultural, and moral ramifications.

A: (by Hummel) Here is a concrete example of what would happen if the public policy issues you raise were discussed in their full ramifications. Let's say a portion of the Florida HIV population were Medicaid eligible—rather than only those with full-blown AIDS. As compelling as Gary Clarke's Florida figures currently are, they would be significantly less optimistic if multiplied by ten, based on the information we have from our TAP center. And there are going to be thousands of people out there who need that kind of access to public health services.

Comment: (by Westmoreland) A General Accounting Office study compared 12 different models for understanding the magnitude of HIV infection, and my sense is that, based on CDC evidence and these other models, we really do know a lot about the extent of infection. But we haven't taken action on what we know.

Q: (by Silverman to Westmoreland) Could you characterize the extent of the HIV epidemic in terms of the population most at risk? Assuming there are a million cases of HIV infection in this country, is the problem predominantly in the poor population?

A: (by Westmoreland) Most people agree that, yes, HIV disproportionately affects the poor at this point. The CDC has done sampling through what they call a "family of surveys"—studies through selected hospitals, prenatal clinics, and sexually-transmitted disease clinics.

However, everyone agrees that we don't know how to model sexual preference because we're working on sexual behavior data from 1948. So both the federal administration and the Congress have stopped attempting to model it.

Comment: (by Hummel) The sero-prevalence data we do have does support the idea that HIV is predominantly infecting minorities. In New Jersey, we did prenatal sero-prevalence testing and found a .5 percent ratio throughout the state. However, in places like Newark, which have a large minority and IV-drug using population, we found a 1.7 to 2 percent ratio. In the Bronx, whole blocks in poor minority neighborhoods are technically totally HIV-infected based on sero-prevalence data.

Q: (by Silverman) That information makes a lot of difference in formulating policy, doesn't it?

A: (by Westmoreland) Yet much the majority of our policy is geared towards a gay, middle-class, white population. We think we've done effective prevention based on the reduced sero-prevalence transmission among middle-class, white gay men. But this reduction may not hold true for minority gay men or for gay men in rural areas. In other words, we're basing current public policy on an epidemic profile from five or six years ago. That means we are essentially writing off the minority population by not developing public policy for their needs.

Q: (by Anderson) What I'm most concerned about is that if we have a million people who are HIV-positive today, how many more will be positive—yet without AIDS—in 1993 to 1995? If you extrapolate a little bit, the numbers become really frightening, and I think we're blind to that.

A: (by Westmoreland) I don't know how we're going to find out the sero-prevalence of HIV in the future. We're hampered by both our lack of knowledge about sexual behavior and our lack of understanding of drug abuse behavior.

I want to caution everyone, though, that if we begin to talk about an HIV epidemic rather than an AIDS epidemic, we may jeopardize the "back-door" access we achieved for people with AIDS in 1984, when presumption of disability made them eligible for Medicaid. If we redefine the spectrum of HIV disease, the Social Security Administration may try to restrain the use of the presumptive disability designation, thus depriving these people of Medicaid.

Q: (by Jones) Haven't treatment costs of other communicable diseases, such as syphilis and gonorrhea, been in the public health budget, rather than charged to a Medicaid or Medicare budget?

A: (by Westmoreland) We have two different programs, I think. Those who come through the EPDST program [Early and Periodic Screening, Diagnosis, and Treatment for children and youth] under Medicaid or through a public hospital clinic would be reimbursed under Medicaid. The other program is the CDC grants program for sexually-transmitted disease control. However, since we now have the highest rate of syphilis in maybe 75 years, these approaches don't appear to be effective models.

Comment: As the son of a chaplain in a tuberculosis sanitorium, it drives me nuts to see that we have not eliminated TB from this country. We don't reimburse well for TB care, and we don't provide for it well through public health programs. Unlike AIDS, we know exactly what to do, yet we've allowed TB to go on existing. And now it's at the highest level in perhaps 25 years.

Q: (by Donley) Have block grant programs had any effect on these problems at all?

A: (by Westmoreland) Perhaps some in maternal and child health and a little bit in the preventive block grant. However, when they were put together in 1981, block grants took a 25 percent cut from the old categorical funding and haven't kept pace with inflation since. So just for pre-AIDS services like hypertension and lead poisoning control, those block grants have been used up.

Q: (by McInturff) There is one effective block grant—the alcohol, drug abuse, and mental health block grant—we're putting a lot of money into drug abuse now. Could you comment on that?

A: (by Westmoreland) It's true that we have put a lot of money into that block grant, but we haven't been able to get any kind of breakdown on how much is going into alcoholism, how much to drug abuse, and how much to mental health—let alone hard versus soft drugs. So we can't answer the question of whether it's helping.

Comment: (by Donley) I would say it's not helping.

Comment: (by Hummel) And its impact on HIV rates or its interrelationship with HIV transmission has been minimal.

Q: (to Hummel and Young) Based on the TAP program, of the 435 participants, 85 percent of those who were asymptomatic HIV patients were already on AZT, meaning they were already hooked into some system of care. What percent of all the people with asymptomatic HIV are being treated in your estimation?

A: (by Young) A lot of physicians were practicing early intervention even before the recommendation to administer early AZT came out. So some patients are receiving early intervention before they enter the TAP program.

A: (by Hummel) One advantage of the TAP program is that we're setting the programs up as resource centers for primary care physicians and other providers. We've developed a state-wide care and treatment protocol. By plugging physicians into TAP centers, we'll begin to get an idea of who is getting what treatment, in what clinical venue. So far no one really knows who is getting the drug or whether it is working.

Q: (by Jones to those who spoke) Are we going to handle AIDS as a separate issue, or are we going to address the AIDS and HIV epidemic—and the treatment issues it raises—through overall restructuring of the health care system?

While ethically it's clear that the HIV epidemic poses urgent problems that must be dealt with immediately, how do we get the needed support politically and tactically? As we all know, the deliberations on AIDS are affected not only by budget analysts looking for cost savings, but also by rigid, uneducated people who don't like folks who are different from them.

My explanation for why more people from Capitol Hill and from the Health Care Financing Administration (HCFA) aren't here today is that they believe that discussing the AIDS issue separately can only go so far. Their present interest is in discussing systems reform, and that isn't all bad. In addition, many people think that the insurance industry has moved counterproductively in choosing to insure only certain categories of people.

The question is, ethically what should we do? But I think we know the answer to that. So the question becomes, politically and practically, where are we going to get the leverage to open up access to health services for people with HIV infection and AIDS?

A: (by Westmoreland) Using the estimates of the Centers for Disease Control, 51 percent of people with HIV infection have T-cell counts of under 500. These people can't wait for systematic reform and national health insurance. Without early intervention, a quarter of these people may be dead by the next congressional session, and half of the survivors may be dead in three to five years. Definitely, structural reforms are needed. But if we wait for systematic reform, we are saying that these people can't have access to health care, and they will die.

Q: (by Jones) Are we as a society going to do what has to be done to intervene for these HIV-infected people? Have we as health care advocates made our case convincingly?

A: (by Westmoreland) The experience is so short with these early intervention drugs that it's almost like planning for delivery of science fiction. But we have to do that. The Florida numbers presented by Gary Clarke are some of the first to show that length of hospital stay was decreased by administration of AZT.

But I think we can make our case by arguing that early intervention postpones spending or actually saves money. This year the Subcommittee on Health and the Environment will be considering access to early intervention drugs for people through Medicaid and through the grant programs.

Comment: (by Hummel) The question actually is two questions. First, are we going to move forward decisively to intervene in this epidemic, or is it going to do us in? I think it's inevitable that, if we sit back and wait, the system will collapse or change in some dramatic way because of the sheer number of people presenting themselves for care.

Second, we must take some very quick, short-range action to create access to care for HIV-infected people. However, we must not separate AIDS and HIV care into a totally different system, because I firmly believe we can create a model of care that is easily transferable. For example, the approach used by the TAP Assessment Centers in New Jersey could be just as applicable to geriatric individuals, to those who have Alzheimer's disease, to those who need long-term care, to those with hemophilia or childhood disabilities—everything.

Comment: (by Young) As Winston Churchill observed, Americans can be counted on to do the right thing—after they've exhausted all other alternatives. An academic policy expert named Charles Lindloom observed that often our policy is made by what he calls "disjointed incrementalism"—or, put more colloquially—muddling through.

What we have now is a number of AIDS-specific strategies, including the Public Health Services programs, and the home and community-based Medicaid waivers that may be AIDS-specific. So the question of whether to have AIDS-specific approaches is somewhat of a straw man.

But we will also have incremental change, or "muddling through." We will find ways to meet the most pressing of the needs of HIV-infected people. And we will continue to debate the issue of how to implement reform. The options of private versus public and direct funding versus insurance mechanisms are critical to this larger debate.

Comment: (by Braslow) I agree that we can't wait for structural reform, and entitlements appear to cost more than anyone thinks they will. But discretionary programs may be a viable option, because they can be repealed when the need is past—as were programs for health professions training, student loans, and health planning.

Comment: (by Clarke) I am worried about urgency, which is what it really comes down to. We must do something about AIDS today, but we must also do something about the larger system tomorrow. For example, in Florida, while 34 percent of hospital days were paid by private insurers in 1987, last year, only 30 percent were. So the gap between what the publics and the privates are paying for is growing. And this is not only for AIDS programs, but for drug abuse and poverty issues, as well. The whole dissolution of society is becoming the burden of a very few institutions.

Comment: (by Jones) As often happens with these conferences, we're coming up with an inclusive answer—that we need to do "all of the above." That is, we must both develop immediate access for HIV-infected people to early intervention services and also work towards changes in the system.

I would also like to comment that with all the great work The Robert Wood Johnson Foundation has done for AIDS, everyone is worried about the Foundation leaving the field at this point. However, we don't want to set up a signal that a foundation shouldn't get into a field because it would be criticized afterwards when it was time to leave. I think that dilemma deserves attention because partnerships between private philanthropy and government must be further explored in the future.

That is my way leading into my thanks to the Foundation and to the other foundations that have stuck their toe in the water on this crucial issue. I do wish more would get in up to their armpits as has The Robert Wood Johnson Foundation.

Closing Statement

Paul S. Jellinek

First of all, I want to take this opportunity to thank all of you for sharing with us what we think has been a very exciting two days.

In particular, I want to acknowledge publicly the pivotal role that our president, Dr. Cluff, has played not only in coming up with the idea for this meeting in the first place, but also in his strong personal support for all of the Foundation's many activities and programs in this very difficult area of AIDS and HIV.

I also want to thank Judy Jones and Karen Matherlee, who together have done such a masterful job in helping us organize this meeting and making it as productive as it has been.

Now, what were we trying to accomplish here?

Well, to put it as simply as I can, what we were trying to do is to bring two very different worlds together—the people out in the field who deliver the services and the people here in Washington who have to think about how to pay for these services.

Why do we think that's worth doing? I guess it's in part because, as Carl Schramm said this morning, we all realize that the way we pay for services ultimately determines the way we deliver them.

So, what has been said over the past two days that might be of use to those of you on the policy side of the process?

First of all, the HIV epidemic is not going away in the foreseeable future, no matter which CDC caseload projection you subscribe to. It is already having a real impact on hospitals—especially public hospitals—and on hospital staffs. Parenthetically, for me probably the most compelling evidence of that impact isn't the statistics that Dennis Andrulis, Chuck Lewis, and Howard Freeman presented yesterday, but rather the high response rates they got to their surveys—and not just from hospitals in New York and San Francisco.

The second thing I think we heard is that there are people in communities all over the country who also are not only willing to respond but who also have actually developed some very creative and important projects that are providing badly needed services. In fact, what has emerged—especially in some of the cities funded under the AIDS Health Services Program and the HRSA program that Judy Braslow described—is a fundamentally new system of community-based care which, as Patricia McInturff told us so eloquently, has potential application well beyond AIDS.

That was the good news.

The downside, I think, is that these new approaches to care are running headlong into a financing system that, again, as Dr. Schramm noted, was designed to pay for acute care. That is what we've spent most of today talking about.

While I may be responsible for this oral summary, there's no way I'm going to try to summarize where we've come out on that complex discussion. We will all have to do that, I think, after the dust has settled and we've had time to do some sifting.

Suffice it to say that the issue of how we pay for AIDS care is inextricably tied to the way we pay for all medical care in this country, and this broader debate over health care financing will probably stretch out for at least as long as Jeff Harris's projections of the AIDS epidemic. The only question I would raise,

Paul S. Jellinek, PhD, is a senior program officer of The Robert Wood Johnson Foundation.

as Tim Westmoreland did, is whether we can afford to wait that long to figure out how to pay for AIDS services that are needed right now.

Let me stop there and again express my thanks to all of you on behalf of the Foundation—not simply for being here, but for actively participating, and through your participation, for helping to bridge the gap between the delivery of frontline services and the formation of the nation's public health policy.

An Overview of AIDS Policy Issues

Policy Considerations For AIDS: A Summary of Key Issues

Deborah E. Lamm, MPA

POLICY CONSIDERATIONS FOR AIDS: A SUMMARY OF KEY ISSUES

Deborah E. Lamm

"The only thing new about AIDS," suggests June Osborn, MD, chair of the National Commission on Acquired Immune Deficiency Syndrome, "is the virus." Neither the medical quandaries, nor financing challenges, nor philosophical dilemmas, nor human inequities exposed by the disease emerge for the first time with AIDS. The clustering of so many issues around AIDS, however, may uniquely embrace significant policy questions that characterize health care in America today.

In the span of less than a decade since AIDS was first identified, the disease has laid claim to many changes. National expenditures have gone from zero to an estimated $4.5 billion for 1991. Whole systems of advocacy and care have sprung up. The person in the street is as likely as not to be conversant with technical jargon such as "exchange of bodily fluids," "AZT," or "HIV." Policies, precautions, and educational tools have been devised which, if followed, could eliminate further spread of the disease. And, more than 70,000 lives have been lost.

Hand in hand with the epidemic have come weighty policy questions.

Absent have been a national strategy for addressing the disease and a financing system responsive to ever-growing needs for services and medical care. Ultimately, all AIDS policy questions come back to these two missing elements. Below are described selected policy concerns stemming from presentations during the workshop.

Data Trends

A slowdown in the rate of AIDS incidence is evident in the period 1987-1989, says Jeffrey Harris, MD, and others. This very good news obscures several related developments.

☐ The slowdown almost certainly reflects a reduction in the incidence of AIDS cases diagnosed only among gay men who do not abuse drugs. This population has consistently made up the largest risk group for the disease, and any changes within it can mask trends among other risk groups. Thus, the seriousness of rising rates of incidence among the relatively smaller numbers of intravenous drug abusers (IVDUs), women and children, and minorities is overshadowed.

☐ Despite the slowdown in the incidence rate, the actual number of new AIDS cases continues to rise. The federal Centers for Disease Control (CDC) projects 296,000 new cases of AIDS in the four-year period 1990 through 1993.

☐ Leveling or reductions in incidence within urban areas hit hardest at the beginning of the epidemic are countered by the appearance of cases or by rising rates of incidence in communities previously spared real impact. For example, in the past year, the annual rate of incidence—number of cases per 100,000 population—has almost quadrupled in Gary, Indiana, from 1.6 to 6.0; it has almost tripled in El Paso, Texas, rising from 2.1 to 6.0.

Deborah E. Lamm, MPA, is the deputy director of The Robert Wood Johnson Foundation's AIDS Prevention and Service Program and formerly served as assistant executive director of the U.S. Conference of Mayors.

☐ In large part due to the identification of drug therapies effective in slowing both the onset of AIDS and progress of the disease, survival rates have improved in the past two years. Over time, says Dr. Harris, the number of people living with AIDS (and HIV-related conditions) will soar. CDC estimates put at 188,000 the number of people who will be living with AIDS in 1993—double the 1989 number of 95,000.

The slowdown in the incidence of AIDS among gay men points to the success of model prevention and education programs devised for this target group. The programs, which were developed in the first wave of high-impact coastal cities, were created essentially by and for a largely educated, salaried, sophisticated, motivated group whose advocacy effectively extended beyond education to raising both public awareness and the first federal and private dollars.

The populations for whom incidence rates are now rising have traditionally been disenfranchised and lacking so-called empowerment, and many are among the 37 million Americans without health insurance. The prospects for advocacy and service delivery for them are daunting. Past efforts in traditional political and health arenas have met with mixed receptivity and uneven success.

Who, for example, speaks for the intravenous drug abuser? Those familiar with AIDS patterns can provide many clinical, rational, and humane reasons for addressing the IVDU-AIDS link. Beyond concerns about the plight of any individual infected with HIV, there are associated societal problems of long-term care costs, spread of HIV to sexual contacts of infected IVDUs and to those with whom needles are shared, and, perhaps most compelling, potential transmission of infection by an HIV-positive pregnant woman to her fetus.

Educational messages fine-tuned for gay men need to be revised to effectively reach IVDUs and other newly emergent high-risk groups. What new approaches will be sponsored, developed, and implemented to reach the IVDU group, whose addiction speaks clearly to the ineffectiveness of traditional public health messages to change behavior? Certainly, a number of possible outreach strategies that are potentially effective may be politically and morally repugnant to some observers and decision makers: Witness the stormy experience of needle-exchange programs, in which addicts can trade in a dirty needle for a clean one. Few such experiments have been tried; some have folded.

The probability of an expanding population living longer with a range of HIV conditions raises questions about what services and support will be available to them. The current health care system is set up to provide acute medical care, leaving those requiring chronic care or non-medical care in a no-man's land.

During the course of the epidemic, countless important programs offering services, support, and care for people with AIDS have blossomed as if by serendipity to meet previously unfilled needs. It is doubtful whether this patchwork of new services surrounding traditional health care services can continue to hold together as the number of people living with AIDS increases. For example, Project Open Hand in San Francisco provides two meals daily to people living with AIDS. Founded in 1985 by Ruth Brinker when she was stunned to discover no such services existed, the program's original seven-person client base is now over 1,500 and growing. The agency's $69,000 budget for 1986 is $3 million in 1990. Still, Ruth Brinker says she is committed to serving all in need and will not put anyone on a waiting list.

Testing

The issue of testing has been explosive since the first marketing of confirmative tests for HIV infection in 1985. Interests initially polarized around the testing issue for as many reasons as there were invested parties.

At the outset, the arguments favoring HIV testing were protecting the national blood supply from infection by contaminated blood and making available information to HIV-positive people who could appropriately modify their lifestyles to prevent infection of others. Some of the arguments against HIV testing were: AIDS activists were wary that testing, either mandatory or voluntary, could leave people vulnerable, and results inappropriately shared could lead to discrimination in housing, jobs, and insurance; and public health departments, already reeling from recent federal cutbacks that had shifted the responsibility for blocks of services to them (in the guise of conversion from categorical to block grants), were disturbed at the prospect of having to provide yet another service—this one with unknown cost implications—since many thought that appropriate informed consent and pre-test and post-test counseling should routinely accompany testing.

In the five years since 1985, many reports, recommendations, and policies have emerged around the testing issue. From the CDC, states, hospital and health associations, public policy and interest groups, and AIDS activist organizations have come a range of protocols—some optional, some binding, some carrying penalties for noncompliance.

Despite these steps, it remains largely the happenstance of where and by whom a test for HIV infection is administered that determines what safeguards, if any, will be in effect. The presence or absence of informed consent, pre-test and post-test counseling, patient confidentiality, or even access to care is irregular in the absence of uniform, mandatory controls.

A 560-hospital study by the University of California at Los Angeles shows that AIDS testing in hospitals is inconsistent among and within institutions:

- [ ] 17 percent of hospitals have no policies governing testing.
- [ ] Many hospitals neither advise patients that they will be (or have been) tested nor provide patients with test results.
- [ ] 40 percent of hospitals never or only sometimes provide pre-test counseling.
- [ ] 25 percent of hospitals transfer patients who test positive for the HIV virus to other institutions.

Alternative drug therapies raised a testing Catch-22. Although drugs such as AZT and aerosol pentamidine had been prescribed for several years to treat advanced cases of AIDS, the discovery that administration of these drugs could effectively delay AIDS symptoms and slow its progress made a persuasive argument for people who might have been exposed to the HIV virus to be tested and tested early. However, until recently, neither Medicaid (the federal/state health insurance program for some poor) nor private health insurance would cover the $1,000 to $6,500 yearly cost of drugs prescribed in preliminary stages of HIV infection because the federal Food and Drug Administration (FDA) had not approved them for this use. Finally, in March 1990, based on two studies, the FDA approved AZT for treating presymptomatic adults infected with HIV.

Because the FDA acted with relative haste in granting this approval, some policy-watchers interpreted the action as determined leadership emerging from the federal government. Others pointed out that questions remain about the availability of AZT and access to it by people who lack insurance. This vital missing piece, on the one hand, along with progress on the other, exemplifies the continued absence of an overall federal strategy to deal with AIDS.

Services and Financing

"There is only recently the recognition that financing drives the delivery system," offers Carl Schramm, President of the Health Insurance Association of America, who believes that the inadequacies of current financing methods are behind the dislocations in this country's health system in general and those of AIDS services in particular. Limitations of the current financing system include, for example:

☐ absence of a good approach to chronic care management
☐ absence of employer coverage for large segments of society
☐ limited availability of alternative treatments
☐ absence of insurance coverage for high-risk people, and
☐ varying levels of access to quality of care.

Many health care financing experts agree that remedying intrinsic service problems requires fundamental reform of the financing systems present in the United States. As to what should be done pending that change, there is less agreement. Should workable interventions be encouraged or be put on hold until needed financial changes are made? Should the growing patchwork of services continue to develop and to be pieced together? Should there be further study? Should drastic financing changes occur now? Should large infusions of dollars be set aside for AIDS-related care and services while, for the present, the remaining care system continues business as usual? Should current definitions of HIV disease be modified from acute to chronic, with minimum service requirements modified as well?

Impact

Across the service continuum are examples of the massive impact that has been brought about by AIDS. Whether isolated by virtue of geographic concentration or representative of a larger picture, the tales are staggering.

First-wave states such as New Jersey and cities such as Dallas have been hard hit. Says Robert Hummel from the New Jersey State Department of Health:

> The large number of asymptomatic HIV-positive individuals, the lack of early intervention programs, and the uneven demographic distribution of the epidemic are creating enormous pressure on state government. Comfortable distinctions between . . . state and federal responsibilities will break down as health systems in high-incidence states approach collapse due to the increasing need for assessment and early intervention.

In agreement is Steven Young, Director of the Care and Treatment Unit within the state's Division of AIDS Prevention and Control, "Systems strained before AIDS/HIV are nearly ready to collapse under the weight of the epidemic." He credits federal and philanthropic dollars with preventing this collapse to date, but he acknowledges the fix is short-term.

In the first years of the AIDS epidemic, Parkland Memorial Hospital in Dallas served as an acute care facility for terminal AIDS patients; now its focus has shifted to chronic care. Case-managed care is provided for 1,300 people monthly in Parkland's outpatient clinic. As these numbers continue to grow, says CEO Ron Anderson, "This will require greater dependence on social services and more need than ever before for case management." Unfortunately, the payment and reimbursement systems remain geared to acute care. As a result, Parkland Memorial annually loses the equivalent of three percent of its total operating budget to treatment of patients with AIDS and HIV.

Across the country, public hospitals are disproportionately impacted by AIDS, with public institutions in the Northeast, in particular, most impacted. Data compiled by the National Public Health and Hospital Institute demonstrate that AIDS patients in hospitals are a low-income, uninsured group. Says study author Dennis Andrulis, "There is a need for the federal government to take a more active role when financing is so critical." Among needed federal interventions identified are: a shift in reimbursement patterns that supports the shift in the locus of care from hospitals to community settings, provision of emergency assistance or impact aid—all in the context of overall changes in the health care system.

Service Program Models

Nationwide, there is a continuum of services responding to the needs of people with AIDS that did not exist 10 years ago. Says Edward N. Brandt, Jr., MD, Director of the AIDS Prevention and Service Program, "We have demonstrated that there is a role in fighting AIDS for every segment of society. In any single community, there is something that can be done by religious organizations, medical groups, public institutions, schools, community agencies, and volunteers."

Many of the model programs, set up to fill gaps, are also redefining AIDS and the needs of people affected by the disease. Various service components extend across successful service models, and some elements of these models are sketched in succeeding paragraphs.

Case Management
Case management is a method of managed care providing coordinated and cohesive access to a full range of health and social services. The Treatment Assessment Program of the State of New Jersey, the Seattle-King County housing program, the housing and long-term care program in Palm Beach County and the Long Island Association for AIDS Care program in Nassau County share an emphasis on linking people to needed AIDS services through case management. Implied in these approaches is a definition of AIDS that is very broad, including HIV-positive, asymptomatic individuals as well as those with more advanced disease. Preliminary evidence from some of these programs demonstrates that managed care reduces hospital admissions and shortens lengths of hospital stay.

Long-range Strategy
An eye toward the future gives many of the models applicability beyond the epidemic. In Seattle-King County, for instance, plans for a new residence for people with AIDS take into account certification requirements for alternative use as a long-term care facility for elderly people.

Community-based Organizations
The leadership and advocacy elements that community-based organizations offer is integral to the success of service programs. Ties to target populations lend legitimacy to efforts of community groups and foster effective outreach.

Volunteers
Volunteers provide service programs with a limitless resource present everywhere, whether they be individual community residents or a group from a specific profession, such as lawyers.

Prevention Programs

Promising preventive interventions are emerging. Public STD clinics in Los Angeles preliminarily have shown that means exist to convey to patients the effectiveness of condom use in lowering STD rates. Program participants exposed to the educational messages developed by the Los Angeles Public Health Foundation are approximately half as likely to return with new STD infections as those who had not received the program messages. Implications of this strategy for reducing HIV infection are apparent. Other prevention programs for migrant workers and inner-city high school students appear to be making headway as well.

Paying for Services

Speaking of the response by private payers to AIDS, Steven Sieverts of Blue Cross/Blue Shield says that these groups treated people with AIDS in much the same way as they treat other ill people. Within the insurance industry, coverage for AIDS-related services is seen as no different—with similar limitations and exclusions—than coverage for other categories of disease-specific services.

The Federal Government

At the federal level, AIDS has been addressed by many agencies, most under the Department of Health and Human Services. The Food and Drug Administration, the National Institutes of Health, the Centers for Disease Control, the Health Resources and Services Administration, and the Health Care Financing Administration all have different funding responsibilities and interests with regard to AIDS. Direction and strategy for these agencies—individually and collectively—have been limited.

A multiyear look at the Health Resources and Services Administration (HRSA) AIDS budget exemplifies the lack of strategy in the federal approach (see chart). Covering more than nine major service areas, the HRSA AIDS budget has more than quadrupled over the five-year period fiscal year (FY) 1986 to projected FY 1991. Only two programs have had long-term stable funding—home health services and subacute care, two programs first set up in FY 1990, which also expire at the end of FY 1990. As a result, there is no request for funding these programs in FY 1991, and no planning for their continuation can take place. Funding levels currently approved by Congress will not meet HRSA operating costs for commitments already in place to 25 sites participating in service demonstration projects. And, while housing needs are severe for people with AIDS, HRSA's facilities' renovation program stems from legislation developed for hospitals; thus a costly and possibly unnecessary medical component must accompany housing program plans considered for support under this revenue source.

The federal government has convened two distinguished AIDS study panels. The President's Commission on Acquired Immune Deficiency Syndrome has completed its work and has made policy recommendations. The independent National Commission on Acquired Immune Deficiency Syndrome has issued two preliminary reports and continues to explore critical questions about AIDS policy, funding, services, and care.

In addition, there are federal studies of far broader application:

☐ Findings of the Pepper Commission/U.S. Bipartisan Commission on Comprehensive Health Care have recently been released. Established in 1988 to examine health insurance reform and long-term care, the panel has recommended a $66 billion program of health insurance and long-term nursing care for those in need. Many questions have resulted from the Commission's report, not the least of which asks where funding is to come from.

☐ The Social Security Advisory Council, a 13-member panel of private-sector experts appointed by HHS Secretary Sullivan, is charged with study of Medicare, Medicaid, and private health care delivery.

Philanthropy

Philanthropy has responded to AIDS by investing primarily in design and demonstration of model programs and systems of care. Since 1985, almost $100 million has come from private sources. However, as Robert Wood Johnson Foundation President Dr. Leighton Cluff notes, private dollars cannot support ongoing systems of care. "The primary role of philanthropy," he says, "is to facilitate the work of others."

HRSA AIDS Program Budget ($ in Millions)

	FY86	FY87	FY88	FY89	FY90	FY91**
Pediatric Service Demonstration Grants	—	—	4.8	7.8	14.8	14.8
Service Demonstration Grants	15.3	10.0	14.4	14.7	17.2	19.4
HIV Services Planning	—	—	—	3.9	—	—
Facilities Construction And Renovation Program	—	—	6.7	3.9	4.3	4.1
Professional Education Programs	—	1.9	11.1	14.6	14.6	21.0
AIDS Drug Reimbursement Program	—	30.0	—	15.0*	29.6	—
Community Health Care Services Program	—	—	—	—	10.8	13.3
Home Health Services	—	—	—	—	19.7	—
Subacute Care Demonstration Projects	—	—	—	—	1.5	—
Total	**15.3**	**41.9**	**37.0**	**59.9***	**112.5**	**72.6**

Plus $5 million contributed by Burroughs-Wellcome Company
**President's Budget.*

Future Considerations

Within the current health care structure, there are pieces that could be independently reformed and reformatted, as has been the practice to date. For example:

☐ Some funding reforms could encourage cost-effective programs. "If I had one policy option to take," says Gary Clarke speaking from his perspective as Assistant Secretary for Medicaid in the State of Florida, "it would be to make an AIDS waiver an optional service under the Medicaid program automatically." He suggests that the case management requirement that accompanies the waiver reaps the double benefit of providing better care at lower cost.

☐ Providers hit with a disproportionate number of AIDS patients could be granted emergency assistance or impact aid. The CARE bill introduced by Senators Edward Kennedy and Orrin Hatch would provide impact aid to a small number of cities with the largest number of reported AIDS cases and emergency assistance to all states to permit development of systematic approaches to handle AIDS. Legislation to direct targeted disaster relief, among other reforms, has been offered in the U.S. Houses of Representatives by Congressman Henry Waxman.

☐ Traditional practices of private payers could change. Early in 1990, for example, The Prudential Insurance Company of America began permitting holders of life insurance policies to obtain most of their benefits if they had been in a nursing home for six months or more, or were likely to die within six months.

☐ AIDS funding in the federal Department of Health and Human Services could be centralized to encourage better planning and management. While recognizing the efficiency of this option, AIDS activists fear the relatively small number of AIDS dollars could be swallowed up in the more massive overall HHS budget.

☐ Conversely, there could be acknowledgement that AIDS is special, thus deserving special funding and services. "This crisis has profound implications for society . . . Somehow this crisis needs to be brought to the attention of our leaders," believes Dr. Edward Andrews, a Robert Wood Johnson Foundation Trustee. Says the Los Angeles Public Health Foundation's Dr. Deborah Cohen, "This is a disease we know how to prevent. We can stop it."

A second major option is to change the structure and financing of health care entirely. According to Dr. Donald Young, Executive Director of the Prospective Payment Assessment Commission, to improve the care of HIV-infected people significantly, this step ultimately must occur. Echoing the thoughts of many health policy analysts who share congressional aide Tim Westmoreland's view that "we can't wait for mandated benefits and minimum health insurance," Dr. Young concedes that the rapid expansion and extremity of needs forces an interim "incremental strategy of 'muddling through.' We will find ways to serve at least the most pressing of those needs. At the same time, though, we will continue to debate the issue of reform." Public officials see the issue of major system reform, he believes, as "far more alive on the agenda today."